RENEWALS 691-4574

DATE DUE

NOV 2 3		
MAY 0 2		
FEB 0 6		SEP 2 1 2000
		NO RENEWALS
FEB 2 6		

Demco, Inc. 38-293

Dangerousness

Dangerousness

Probability and prediction, psychiatry and public policy

Edited by

CHRISTOPHER D. WEBSTER
MARK H. BEN-ARON
STEPHEN J. HUCKER

Clarke Institute of Psychiatry
and
University of Toronto

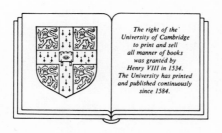

The right of the
University of Cambridge
to print and sell
all manner of books
was granted by
Henry VIII in 1534.
The University has printed
and published continuously
since 1584.

CAMBRIDGE UNIVERSITY PRESS

Cambridge
London   New York   New Rochelle
Melbourne   Sydney

Published by the Press Syndicate of the University of Cambridge
The Pitt Building, Trumpington Street, Cambridge CB2 1RP
32 East 57th Street, New York, NY 10022, USA
10 Stamford Road, Oakleigh, Melbourne 3166, Australia

First published 1985

Printed in the United States of America

Library of Congress Cataloging in Publication Data
Main entry under title:
Dangerousness: probability and prediction, psychiatry
  and public policy.
Based on a series of lectures delivered during the 1981–82 academic year
  at the Clarke Institute of Psychiatry in Toronto.
Includes index.
1. Forensic psychiatry – North America – Addresses,
essays, lectures.   2. Violence – Prediction – North
America – Addresses, essays, lectures.   3. Preventive
detention – North America – Addresses, essays, lectures.
I. Webster, Christopher D., 1936–   .   II. Ben-Aron,
Mark H. III. Hucker, Stephen J.   [DNLM: 1. Commitment
of Mentally Ill.   2. Crisis Intervention.   3. Forensic
Psychiatry.   4. Mental Disorders – diagnosis.   5. Prognosis.
6. Public Policy.   7. Violence.   WM 33.1 D182]
RA1151.D26 1985   364'.41   84–20059
ISBN 0 521 30029 0

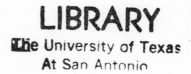

Contents

Tables and figures

Tables

vii

Figures

Contributors

Mark H. Ben-Aron Staff Psychiatrist in Charge, Forensic Inpatient Unit, Clarke Institute of Psychiatry; Assistant Professor of Psychiatry, University of Toronto

Bernard M. Dickens Professor, Faculty of Law, Centre of Criminology and Faculty of Medicine, University of Toronto

Park Elliott Dietz Associate Professor of Law and of Behavioral Medicine and Psychiatry, School of Law, University of Virginia

Donald G. Dutton Associate Professor of Psychology, University of British Columbia

Cyril Greenland Professor, School of Social Work, Associate, Department of Psychiatry, McMaster University

R. Brian Haynes Associate Professor, Department of Clinical Epidemiology and Biostatistics, Department of Medicine, McMaster University

Stephen J. Hucker Chief of Forensic Service, Clarke Institute of Psychiatry; Associate Professor of Psychiatry, University of Toronto

Barry A. Martin Head, Epidemiology and Biostatistics Research Section and Staff Psychiatrist, Clarke Institute of Psychiatry; Assistant Professor of Psychiatry, University of Toronto

Virginia J. McFarlane, University of Toronto

Robert J. Menzies Instructor, Department of Criminology, Simon Fraser University

Diana S. Sepejak Senior Research Officer, Ontario Ministry of Correctional Services

Henry J. Steadman Director, Special Projects Research Unit, New York State Office of Mental Health

ix

Alan A. Stone Professor of Law and Psychiatry in the Faculty of Law and the Faculty of Medicine, Harvard University

Christopher D. Webster Research Scientist, Metropolitan Toronto Forensic Service, Clarke Institute of Psychiatry; Professor of Psychiatry, Psychology and Criminology, University of Toronto

Foreword

In recent years, in most parts of the world, there has been a surge of interest in the discipline that has come to be called "forensic psychiatry." The British Royal College of Psychiatrists has a section of forensic psychiatry with an increasing membership; in England and Wales there is a government-sponsored development program for "security units"; in the United States of America there is the growing American Academy of Psychiatry and the Law; and the United States is moving toward specialist board examinations in forensic psychiatry. The same trends are also evident in Canada with its network of regional psychiatric centers for mentally abnormal offenders and its growing provincial programs. Most of the growth, however, has involved service developments: reports to courts, assessment of security, long-term hospitalization, and advice to prison authorities. Academic developments, especially research, have lagged behind. A discipline that devotes most of its effort to the provision of services and too little to research will ossify, wither, and eventually die. Let us hope that this fate does not befall forensic psychiatry, for the mentally abnormal offender patient is in urgent need of better care and attention in all parts of the world.

This volume is evidence that others share my concern. The book springs from a lively center of academic forensic psychiatry at the Clarke Institute of Psychiatry in Toronto. The editors and authors have addressed a major contemporary issue in North America: dangerousness. I say North America for it is my impression that the subject of dangerousness looms larger there than elsewhere. Certainly, dangerousness is a matter of some debate in the United Kingdom, with its indeterminate sentences, special hospitals, and prison parole board. Furthermore, an influential English book on the topic has been produced by Jean Floud and Warren Young (*Dangerousness and Criminal Justice*, London: Heinemann, 1981). But the subject does not seem to have the preoccupying power in the United Kingdom that it has in North America. Perhaps it should. If my impression is correct, this in itself is of academic interest, and a comparative study could perhaps shed some light on the fundamental nature of the problem. But that is for the future and the subject of another book. In the meantime, this volume will inform interested readers both within and outside of North America about the dilemma of dangerousness.

The volume clearly sets out the nature of the problem. Most of the arguments for and against the use of psychiatry as a predictive and a coercive discipline are rehearsed, and we learn, yet again, that our ability to forecast which people will do harm in the future is very poor. I like Professor Stone's exhortation that we stick to short-term predictions. I like Professor Greenland's view that prediction should be a dynamic rather than a static art, and I very much share his enthusiasm for increased research endeavor. Perhaps future research could concentrate on the management and treatment of violent patients in a flexible setting to show how effective or ineffective psychiatric intervention can be. Dr. Dietz's chapter should be read by all forensic psychiatrists, for it not only sets up some neat and testable hypotheses and makes a plea for better training, but also clearly emphasizes that the area of greatest concern to the psychiatrist should be the patient who has committed grave harm – common ground with the Floud and Young report. Perhaps much of the confusion in this field is due to muddle about the kinds of behaviors that are being predicted and/or prevented. Dr. Steadman's contribution raises all sorts of questions in my mind about the perception many of us have, and which his data refute, that prisons are taking more disturbed individuals than they used to.

Every chapter is worth reading and raises interesting questions. Such is the hallmark of a good academic book. It is now up to all of us in this field, whatever our background discipline, to inquire further, collect more data, and debate actively.

JOHN GUNN
Professor of Forensic Psychiatry
Institute of Psychiatry
University of London

Acknowledgments

This volume had its origin in a series of lectures sponsored by the Metropolitan Toronto Forensic Service, the Clarke Institute of Psychiatry, the Law Foundation of Ontario, and the Department of Psychiatry of the University of Toronto. We are most grateful for the financial support received from these institutions. The lectures were delivered during the 1981–2 academic year and were attended by forensic clinicians as well as colleagues in law and corrections. The original lectures have been reworked into written form, and the editors are most grateful to the contributors for taking so much trouble over their manuscripts. Our thanks are due to Mrs. Kim Yoshiki of METFORS for typing the manuscripts so patiently and so ably. As well, we thank the staff at Cambridge University Press, particularly Susan Milmoe, Editor, Behavioral Sciences, and Mary Nevader, who copyedited the manuscript very carefully and capably.

C.D.W.
M.H.B.-A.
S.J.H.

Introduction

*Christopher D. Webster, Mark H. Ben-Aron,
and Stephen J. Hucker*

In a previous volume that we edited entitled *Mental Disorder and Criminal Responsibility* (Hucker, Webster, & Ben-Aron, 1981), Sir Martin Roth remarked: "To make a significant impression upon criminal violence and dangerous anti-social behaviour in society might take decades or longer. A bold and ambitious start should, therefore, be made on this task" (p. 109). It was this kind of statement that convinced us that our next work should be on the "dangerousness issue."

The prediction of dangerous behavior has become a central topic in psychiatry during recent years. Research studies have called into serious question the ability of mental health professionals to predict the dangerous behavior of their clients, and there have been many patients, relatives, and professionals whose lives have been affected by recent key legal rulings on issues related to the prediction of dangerous behavior. Monahan, in his book *Predicting Violent Behavior* (1981), would seem to have made something of that "bold and ambitious start" called for by Sir Martin. The book, which summarizes ably the present state of knowledge about the prediction of violent behavior, has been very well received. Its success derives partly from the fact that it offers a readable and informed survey of the literature but more importantly from the fact that it provides a model, a way of looking at the issues. Above all, it suggests courses of action. These courses of action are the more interesting because – and this is a point seized on by Cyril Greenland in the present volume – the author, John Monahan, has himself altered his outlook over several years of careful study of the problem. On the one hand, he recognizes the very grave scientific, ethical, and legal problems involved in predicting violent behavior, but on the other, he sees that, at least in some cases, the clinician may feel obligated to offer his or her services to the court. We sympathize with this view, and the present material has been collected and arranged accordingly.

In his book, Monahan (1981) says that "one would have to be completely out of touch with recent developments in criminal and mental health law not to notice that the prediction of violent behavior by mental health professionals has been

1

under sustained attack'' (pp. 26–7). He goes on to point out that there have been three main criticisms: (a) that it is scientifically impossible to predict dangerous behavior; (b) that, even if it were shown to be possible to make accurate forecasts, it would curtail the civil liberties of patients and prisoners; and (c) that mental health professionals should not attempt such prediction because it interferes with their traditional helping role. Monahan correctly notes that the professional attack on prediction has been led by Professor Alan Stone and that Stone's (1975) monograph, *Mental Health and the Law: A System in Transition,* has had highly influential effects.

The present volume starts appropriately with a new contribution from Alan Stone. In this chapter Stone advances with considerable force the important points outlined by Monahan. With respect to the empirical argument, he tells us, ''Listening to a lot of irrelevant and perhaps false information does not improve one's ability to make predictions.'' He is of the view that published studies on the prediction of dangerous behavior have been ''woefully inadequate, poorly conceived, wrongly interpreted, and well below any acceptable standard of scientific research or even solid clinical experience.'' With respect to the civil liberties argument, he says: ''If the patient is dangerous but has committed no crime, the patient cannot morally be confined on any theory of punishment. What we then confront is the preventive detention decision, and it derives not from jurisprudence but from prudence alone.'' With respect to the idea that mental health professionals should not allow their energies to be siphoned off by attempts to do something they cannot do (i.e., predict dangerousness) but should rather get on with what they can do (i.e., treat the mentally disordered), he remarks, ''As psychiatrists our essential policy should be to emphasize our therapeutic function, to put our patients first whenever we can, and to repudiate the police role whenever possible.'' These three arguments are not the only ones Professor Stone uses to make the point that the prediction of dangerous behavior is an ''empirical quicksand'' and that psychology and psychiatry should get clear of it as expeditiously as possible. These ideas, so eloquently expressed here, offer an obvious challenge and must be considered deeply by any student interested in prediction and public policy issues.

Professor Greenland acknowledges at the outset that in trying to deal with violence and mental disorder we are tackling something that ''has plagued humankind since the dawn of history'' and that difficulties associated with this problem ''are unlikely to be solved by semasiological juggling or by modern technology.'' He goes on to imply that the major studies on the prediction of dangerousness, although provoking greatly needed research and thinking, may have had considerable methodological faults. These studies, because of their essentially negative findings, might have cast too dark a shadow on clinical practice. He then points out that ''in the absence of publically acceptable alternatives psychiatrists will continue to be called on by the courts to predict dangerousness or by parole boards or advisory review boards to determine if and when a dangerous offender is fit to be returned to the community." He tells psychiatrists to "stop being apologetic and defensive and strive to improve their skills in this difficult and contentious area." Cyril Greenland writes not only as a researcher, but also as a clinician. He is interested in the phenomenology of violence associated with mental illness and draws on his own studies to tell us something about that phenomenology. Toward the end of his chapter he remarks that further progress in forensic psychiatry will "depend . . . on the ability of psychiatrists to accept the offender fully as a person and recognize the connections between his or her murderous impulses and the experience of economic, political, and psychological powerlessness." The idea expressed in this sentence provides a nearly perfect springboard for the chapter by Christopher Webster and Mark Ben-Aron that follows.

Webster and Ben-Aron attempt in chapter 3 a speculative essay based on a piece of literature. This continues a tradition begun in our earlier work in which Margaret Webster pointed to Dostoyevsky's ability in *Crime and Punishment* to examine Raskolnikov's state of mind in such a way as to cast light on issues related to criminal and personal responsibility. It was her contention, one we followed, that the descriptive and analytic powers of novelists can sometimes be brought to bear on key problems in forensic psychiatry. After some thought, we fixed on the characters of Doctor Fischer and Jones from one of Graham Greene's novels. This story gave us a chance to follow up Cyril Greenland's conviction that it is naive as well as useless to assume that the impulse to rape or kill "resides like a malignancy within an individual." Greenland argues for an assessment process that is not "static" and insists that dangerous offenders themselves be included in research projects. In our essay we are interested in the way in which Mr. Greene deals with the relationship between assessor and assessee and how he draws out very delicately the point that those who wish to understand a dangerous individual should begin by taking a good look at themselves. We treat the Greene novel as a "case study." Some readers will, we hope, like our essay. Others can seek solace in the more mainstream statistical and legal studies that follow.

It was our thought from the first that many forensic psychiatrists and other specialists do not know nearly enough about the basic statistics necessary for an understanding of the controversies in the field. Because almost every paper published on the psychiatric prediction of dangerousness mentions "the false positive problem," few can escape learning what a false positive is. But the contemporary reader requires a somewhat deeper knowledge to appreciate some of the niceties of design and interpretation. It was for this reason that we turned to an epidemiologist, Brian Haynes. His chapter makes it clear that unreliability among clinicians exists in many areas of medicine, that such unreliability is to be expected, and that it can be reduced, sometimes quite simply. He reminds us that we shall likely be better off with an assessment device that, even though somewhat unreliable, measures something important, rather than with a measure of a trivial event that might have been recorded with great precision and reliability. In his words, "Thus, one might distinguish between what is important to measure and what one can measure well." He suggests that clinicians are almost encouraged to be vague and noncommittal in giving prognoses and that they must be trained to be more systematically critical about their clinical skills. His comments about clinical decision making apply directly to the assessment and prediction of dangerous behavior. He makes the point that all we can ever hope to deal with are probabilities and infers that we can hardly expect to improve our predictive powers until we establish what our predictive base rates actually are. The technology is available. What we need is a greater emphasis on critical self-appraisal of clinical activity.

Dr. Barry Martin, in chapter 5, takes up where Haynes leaves off. He reminds us that "the critical examination of error remains a cornerstone of continuing medical education to improve diagnostic accuracy." Martin acknowledges at the outset the fact that, broadly, inter-rater diagnostic agreement among psychiatrists tends to be disappointing and disconcertingly low. One reason for this, or so he argues, is that "for some mental disorders a medical diagnosis is nothing more than an artifact of the overinclusiveness of the field of psychiatry." He offers a succinct summary of main findings from most of the older, well-established studies but concentrates his attention on recent advances in the use of standardized clinical examinations and on the *Diagnostic and Statistical Manual of Mental Disorders,* 3rd ed. (DSM III) (1980) of the American Psychiatric Association. In the course of a description of the main categories in DSM III, he notes that the antisocial personality classification is of special interest to forensic clinicians. Yet, despite his guarded enthusiasm for DSM III generally, he points out that "the global term 'antisocial personality' is of much less predictive usefulness than is the precise itemization of the antisocial behaviors and their temporal sequence to determine whether there has been a progressive escalation of severity or whether a particular behavior is a sporadic or isolated event." This notion strikes us as being very important indeed. We need, in forensic psychiatry, to develop a specially constructed classificatory system based on new measures. Although this may indeed be a good idea, we should not lose sight of one of Martin's concluding comments, namely, that clinicians are often inexcusably lax in employing the carefully worked-out systems they already have. Using his own observations, he shows that clinicians all too often fail to determine whether a patient really does meet the DSM III or other such criteria for a mental disorder. When structured interview and psychological tests are available and called for, they frequently are not applied, and if the criteria require follow-up examinations over a period to determine the amount and rate of behavioral or other change, they usually are not met. This leads him to conclude that, although we have in hand more solid research findings on reliability than most people realize, we face a huge problem in persuading clinicians to regiment themselves properly in their vital everyday work. Perhaps for the title of this book we should have included not just "public policy" but also "professional policy."

In chapter 6 Park Dietz follows Dr. Martin in trying to draw the attention of clinicians to "remediable errors." He points to the amount and kind of data that ought to be collected in the course of an attempt to assess an individual's propensity for dangerous behavior (interviews with living victims of current and past offenses, visits to crime scenes, etc). The list is extensive and causes Dietz to note that "in practice, this complete range of sources of information is almost never consulted." Of course, it takes time and money to be so thorough, yet, as he points out, the costs are actually no greater than in some medical and surgical evaluations. Opinions about "dangerousness," when formed on the basis of cursory examinations, can sometimes set in motion extremely formal, protracted, and expensive court hearings, to say nothing about the unnecessary and debilitating confinement of prisoners and patients. Dr. Dietz argues that most of the evaluations of dangerousness published to date are based on flimsy or inappropriate predictive work and is led to charge, "Judging our clinical predictive capacities on the basis of outcomes for inmates discharged from institutions for the criminally insane is like evaluating current medical technology on the basis of the infant mortality rate in Third World countries."

The core of Dietz's chapter is devoted to an original attempt to create some predictive hypotheses. He establishes, albeit tentatively and with much qualification, a scheme that identifies first-, second-, and third-rank predictors. The idea is that some "intolerable crimes" are more predictable than others. First-rank predictors (e.g., one murder with cannibalism) are more powerful than second-rank predictors (e.g., sadistic sexual fantasies and a history of any violent felony), which in turn are more powerful than predictors of the third rank (e.g., age 16–24). This is an intriguing thought, and we are not aware of any other attempts to conceptualize the issues in this way. Dietz has specified both his theory and the predictor variables in considerable detail, pointing out that the hypothesis is largely testable (although he does note that, in strictly practical terms, "customary forms of research are not possible for some hypothesized predictors, because individuals known to have these features are usually incarcerated for lengthy periods"). He is here referring especially to those predictors of the first rank. As it turns out, however, first-rank predictors are "so obvious" that this is not necessarily a serious impediment to future research. Dietz actually goes farther than this in noting that third-rank predictors are "so weak" that they correspond to what in conventional psychiatric terms we call "soft signs." This leads him to a conclusion that could have a specific influence on the design of future research studies. He says, "The task for clinicians and researchers is to identify, verify, and articulate to policy makers the nature and probabilistic importance of predictors. Second-rank predictors have the highest priority for this work." In more general terms, Dietz is attempting to make us aware of the fact that psychiatrists, psychologists, and other mental health workers do not know much about predicting violent behavior, that they are not trained for the job, and that they make little effort to acquire the requisite formal knowledge and experience. The formal knowledge lies, so he argues, in the domain of clinical criminology. It is his view that "psychiatrists and psychologists who have no knowledge of crime have no more business predicting crime than other citizens."

Training is the point of engagement for Donald Dutton in chapter 7. He shows how it might be possible, following Barry Martin's line of thought, to develop specific diagnostic tests for use in the assessment and prediction of dangerous behavior. Wife assault is the specific focus of his attention. After offering a new theory that centers on the concepts of intimacy and power, he describes his own recently developed videotape scenes portraying different kinds of marital disharmony. These tapes are shown to husbands convicted of assaults on their wives. Dr. Dutton hopes that, aside from pinpointing more precisely the causes of wife battering, these kinds of carefully constructed tapes will eventually become "standardized tests with broader utility in the assessment of violence potential and of sexual violence potential in particular." Put simply, if a man is apt to become violent in the home, it makes obvious sense to concentrate attention on what lies behind commonly occurring marital squabbles. This is a general approach called for by Monahan (1981) when he says, "One novel method of assessing the effect of environmental variables upon violent behavior is to assess a person in terms of the characteristics of the environments in which he or she becomes violent" (p. 140). Dutton reports, on the basis of preliminary exploration, some success in getting men to identify and record the situations in which they lose control. Dutton's work can best be thought of as an attempt at the kind of "ecological" theory called for by Monahan (1981, p. 130) and Menzies, Webster, and Sepejak in chapter 8.

The idea that accuracy of prediction could be enhanced by paying closer attention to the contextual determinants of dangerous behavior is one of several conclusions reached by Robert Menzies, Christopher Webster, and Diana Sepejak in chapter 8. The investigators report the results of a major study in which clinicians made predictions about a large number of people ordered for brief assessment by the courts. Patient records were searched after a 2-year interval, and predictions were correlated with outcomes. The size of these correlations varied according to professional discipline, individual clinician, and type of patient. Although many of the correlations were statistically significant, they tended to be low by conventional standards. The authors, however, are at some pains to point out that it may not be surprising that such correlations mainly fail to exceed the .40 "sound barrier." They note several methodological complexities in conducting research on the capacity of clinicians to predict dangerous behavior and insist that these issues be tackled. As they say, "The onus is emphatically on practitioners and researchers to demonstrate this capacity," and "In the absence of ethical, theoretical, and empirical support, psychiatry may indeed be performing a spurious and arbitrary control function."

Henry Steadman, who with Joseph Cocozza established a personal research career initially on the basis of the extraordinary book *Careers of the Criminally Insane* (1974), offers us in chapter 9 the bare bones of a new piece of research still in progress. Like his earlier work, this is concerned with the career patterns of institutionalized people. He refers here to "confinement careers" and deals with two main groups; those who enter prisons and those who enter mental hospitals. The study is a longitudinal one that explores the characteristics of individuals admitted to both the correctional and mental health systems in 1968 and 1978. Data come from records obtained in six states. The point is to establish whether the jails are, over time, becoming increasingly populated by mental patients and whether the hospitals are accepting more and more people with criminal proclivities. This forecasting is, of course, on a much broader scale than that attempted by Menzies et al. in the previous chapter.

Dr. Barry Martin shares Henry Steadman's interest in examining fluctuations in the number of people entering and leaving the mental health system. In chapter 10 he provides evidence to suggest that "although there has been a dramatic increase in the total rate of admission in the past few decades, expressed as a rate per unit of population, admissions for the severe mental disorders (psychoses) have remained relatively constant over time." He infers that, although the legislators are occasionally impelled to alter the wording of civil commitment statutes, the actual practices of doctors change little in response to these legal maneuverings. As he says, "The clinical decision-making process would appear to be independent of legislation." He is stating in different words a remark attributed to a knowledgeable physician by Dr. W. O. McCormick, one of the lecturers in the series on which this book is based. The comment as cited by McCormick (1981) was, "Doctors will continue to certify those whom they really believe should be certified; they will merely learn a new language" (p. 717). This brings us to the heart of a problem central to Martin's chapter and indeed this volume. How is it possible to write from a legal point of view sufficiently precise criteria for committing individuals civilly or declaring them "dangerous offenders" and, at the same time, to provide a mechanism to ensure that the particular case accords with those stated definitions? Martin himself says, "The most precise definition is of little use if there are no valid, or at least reliable, means of determining the degree of concordance between the facts of a case and the definition."

There are other problems raised by Martin. He argues that, whereas the criminal justice system is in the main concerned with events that have happened in the past, the process of civil commitment procedure is designed to deal with anticipated behavior. It is, as he says, an instrument for preventive detention, and because of this he suggests that there "is a clear limitation to the extent to which one may apply legal concepts of due process to civil commitment." This is an interesting thought, which he follows up by suggesting that, although on the surface it seems as if the criminal justice procedures can be fairly grafted to civil commitment practice, any real correspondence between the two applications is more or less spurious. The real trouble, so Martin argues, is that the issues go beyond law and beyond medicine. He tells us, "The current medicolegal impasse with respect to the criteria for civil commitment will not be resolved unless the social considerations are more fully appreciated." As social architects tighten and refine the civil commitment criteria under law (and no doubt precisely the same could be said about dangerous offender legislation), it is easy to shift the grounds for commitment or indefinite incarceration more definitely into the domain of "dangerousness." But as Martin points out, with considerable reference to Alan Stone's writings, this may not be very wise given the published predictive performance of modern mental health workers.

Martin leaves us with the firm impression that, although beguiling to think otherwise, there can never be a completely satisfactory test for use in civil commitment proceedings. Perhaps it is, to use a metaphor that comes to mind after reading his chapter, like trying to put up single-handedly a tent in a high wind. There is the law at one corner, psychiatry at another, the patient at a third, and civil liberties groups at the fourth. It is easy enough to get one corner established, a little harder to get two, quite difficult to get three, and just about impossible to get the fourth in place. But the real trouble is that it is society as a whole that makes the wind blow, and the wind is very changeable. All the same, it is probably more sensible to try to erect a tent under difficult circumstances than simply to lie down and be enveloped by the elements.

Bernard Dickens opens his analysis of legal and policy issues with reference to the *Tarasoff* case. He is interested not only in the case itself, but in the way professional groups, such as the American Psychiatric Association and the American Psychological Association, have recently responded to the charge that the prediction of dangerous behavior lies largely beyond present clinical competence. He suggests that "the disclaimer may render unworkable not only liability under the broad *Tarasoff* principle, but several legal institutions that have become based on the belief, once encouraged by mental health professionals, that they possess the professional skill generally to predict dangerousness.'' *Tarasoff* poses a major challenge to mental health professionals in that, if they want to be excused from legal liability for failing to predict dangerous behavior accurately, they must define their competence to exclude that predictive skill. Of course, this of necessity restricts the scope of practice and expert status. On the one hand, the professions can, by circumscribing their roles, protect themselves to some extent against demands of competence that cannot be fulfilled. On the other hand, *Tarasoff* and other related cases notwithstanding, the courts continue to depend heavily on expert testimony in several areas bearing on issues of predicting dangerous behavior. In Canada, for example, the law demands that at least two psychiatrists testify under the dangerous offender legislation. Professor Dickens points out that the dangerous offender legislation permits criminologists (and psychologists) to testify *in addition to* psychiatrists. Nonetheless, it would appear that the law views criminologists as being less qualified than psychiatrists or psychologists. But, as Dickens argued, ''Ironically, they may be the 'other professionals,' whose predictions have been judicially recognized to be more accurate.''

Dickens does not argue, however, that the powers once vested in psychiatry should be promptly turned over to clinical criminologists or other such professionals. After a penetrating analysis of the influence of the various mental health professions in several key areas related to the prediction of dangerousness, and after showing how this influence has changed in recent years partly as a result of scientific studies and partly as a result of legal rulings, he opts to place the responsibility squarely with the courts. He urges ''(a) that 'dangerousness' be recognized as a legal status as opposed to a psychiatric condition and (b) that dangerousness be determined by due process of law in adequately conducted hearings.'' He then shows how extant legal models could be adapted to deal with dangerousness issues including civil commitment. His analysis takes note of the fact that this ''judicialization of civil committal'' might sometimes interfere with mental health care and treatment and that mental health professionals might spend more, not less, time in court. He sees no real alternative to this state of affairs, however, given the fact that mental health professionals apparently do not have the means to predict dangerous behavior in individual cases and given the basic premise that individuals should not be obliged to give up their liberty without full protection from due process.

Virginia McFarlane introduces her chapter by explaining that she had the misfortune to be a student in one of the senior editor's classes. In this role she found herself assigned the task of reading a final draft of the present book along with various other books and papers on the topic of dangerousness. Rather than simply regurgitate this material, she chose to organize her opinions in an unusual and interesting fashion. Here, she selects a position, one reasonably close, as it turns out, to that of the present editors, and conducts a spirited argument through an imaginary lawyer hired to defend clinicians formally on trial. McFarlane's judge concludes, "Mental health professionals are, and will be, the best individuals for the jobs of predicting dangerousness and rendering such predictions as expert testimony in court." Although the chapter contains some new ideas and makes reference to several papers not considered by the other authors, it is best viewed as an addendum. The real conclusion of the volume is Bernard Dickens' contribution.

We have deliberately structured this volume with medically trained, legally knowledgeable Professor Stone at the beginning and legally trained, medically knowledgeable Professor Dickens toward the end. Starting with different premises and working from different areas of scholarship, they reach much the same general conclusion: Psychiatry and the other mental health disciplines must accept the fact that they can presently claim only limited ability to predict the dangerous behavior of their patients. This being the case, both authors argue for shifting the balance of decision-making power to the legal domain. Stone argues that the involvement of psychiatry in determining dangerousness does nothing but weaken the profession's credibility. Dickens points out that psychiatry probably cannot have it both ways forever; that is, the discipline cannot accept the responsibility for dangerousness determinations without putting up the evidence that it "has the goods."

In the nine chapters that separate Professor Stone and Professor Dickens, our distinguished authors suggest to mental health professionals and researchers what they must try to do if they are to alter the status quo. There can be little question that, with proper attention to research considerations, psychiatrists and their colleagues in related disciplines could do much to improve their image in this area of scientific endeavor. Monahan (1981) has given many suggestions about the form that new research might take, and our contributors have developed some of these and offered others. It is not that we lack ideas or the ability to articulate them. What we need is implementation and careful study. Even though such work cannot necessarily overcome conceptual difficulties that *at present* seem more or less intractable, a strong case can be made for doing what lies before us. Lawyers and judges are remarkably good, or so it would appear, at reading the scientific literature when it suits their interest or convenience (Appelbaum, 1984) and because their reading and opinion affect crucially the development of legal custom and the preparation of new legislation, mental health workers, researchers, and patient-prisoners themselves can only hope that the courts in the future will become increasingly willing to accept the outcome from properly ordered scientific studies on prediction issues rather than, as at present, generally unsubstantiated professional opinions.

References

Appelbaum, P. S. The Supreme Court looks at psychiatry. *American Journal of Psychiatry, 1984, 141,* 827–35.

Diagnostic and statistical manual of mental disorders (3rd ed.). Washington, D.C.: American Psychiatric Association, 1980.

McCormick, W. O. Involuntary commitment in Ontario: Some barriers to the provision of proper care. *Canadian Medical Association Journal, 1981, 124,* 715–17.

Monahan, J. *Predicting violent behavior: An assessment of clinical techniques.* Beverly Hills: Sage, 1981.

Roth, M. Modern psychiatry and neurology and the problem of responsibility. In S. J. Hucker, C. D. Webster, & M. H. Ben-Aron (Eds.), *Mental disorder and criminal responsibility.* Toronto: Butterworths, 1981.

Steadman, H. J., & Cocozza, J. J. *Careers of the criminally insane.* Lexington, Mass.: Heath, 1974.

Stone, A. A. *Mental health and the law: A system in transition.* Washington, D.C.: U.S. Government Printing Office, 1975.

1 The new legal standard of dangerousness: fair in theory, unfair in practice

Alan A. Stone

On November 17, 1981, John Ashbrook, a U. S. representative from the state of Ohio, had printed in the Congressional Record the following statement: Psychiatrists "have as much understanding of the human mind as the butcher, the baker and the candlestick maker." He likened the psychiatrist to the "bogeyman." In the same vein, the attorney general of Massachusetts commented on a case of a patient who had been released from a state hospital and murdered a child. He told the press, "Psychiatrists know about as much as witch doctors." "Bogeyman" and "witch doctor" seem rather extreme terms, particularly when we in the psychiatric profession have a sense that psychiatry has moved into a new scientific era. How should we understand these criticisms from the law? Is this just the same old legal antagonism to psychiatry that peaked in the 1970s, fueled by critics like Dr. Szasz, who said there is no such thing as mental illness? I think not. Rather, I would suggest that we have now entered a second generation of insults against psychiatry and legal dissatisfaction with it. My explanation of these second-generation phenomena is closely related to the theme of this volume.

The first generation of legal reform attacked the ideology of psychiatry with its medical model and replaced it with a legal procedural approach. This approach required psychiatrists to do what we are *unable* to do: to predict violence, to prognosticate future behavior. It is our failure to do what we cannot do that has led to this second generation of criticism and a new wave of legal reform.

In what follows, I discuss the legal problems of dangerousness in three sections. First, I deal with the American criminal justice system itself; second, I discuss future dangerousness as a criterion for capital punishment in the United States; and third, I comment on the relevance of the legal standard of dangerousness to civil commitment.

13

The Anglo-American criminal justice system

During the past two decades, the question of dangerousness, the clinical and statistical prediction of violent behavior (which forms the content of the following chapters), has become the chief battlefield in the struggle between law and psychiatry. It was my own view from the very beginning of my work in these two disciplines that this was the wrong battlefield on which psychiatry should try to take a stand. My review of the prediction literature, both statistical and clinical, convinced me that we had no solid empirical grounds for making anything more than very short term predictions of violent behavior. By ''short term'' I mean evaluating the patient's current mental status and estimating how long that mental status will continue.

I found the published studies of prediction woefully inadequate, poorly conceived, wrongly interpreted, and well below any acceptable standard of scientific research or even solid clinical experience. Parenthetically, I note that psychiatric research on the basic subject of violence, even separate from the problem of prediction, leaves much to be desired.

But it was not because we know so little (and still do) that I thought dangerousness was the wrong battlefield for psychiatry. I had become convinced that our critics were correct in one very important theme, namely, that our profession had become involved in a series of complicated double-agent roles. We were functioning, on the one hand, as therapists with our central responsibility directed to the patient and with the public conception of our role shaped in that way. But at the same time, at least in the United States, we had begun increasingly to function as agents of social control. Particularly I would emphasize that we are asked to serve as police officers whose responsibility it is to protect society, the family, and other institutions against the patient.

This is not the occasion to unravel the complexities of double agentry. I emphasize only the conflict between our therapeutic and police roles. I have argued previously that as psychiatrists our essential policy should be to emphasize our therapeutic function, to put our patients first whenever we can, and to repudiate the police role whenever possible. Treatment, I argue, should be the basic domain of the mental health system. Protection of society should be the basic domain of the criminal justice system. This is the fundamental policy principle I have urged on the psychiatric establishment. It should be the animating spirit of the legal reforms in civil commitment, the right to treatment and the right to refuse treatment, the least restrictive alternative, and it should apply at all the junctures between psychiatry and the criminal law as I have tried to argue in my own writing (e.g., Stone, 1976, 1981). Unfortunately, until recently, in most of these areas the courts have not been receptive to therapeutic criteria and therapeutic standards. Instead, they have imposed on psychiatry at every place of conflict between the roles of therapist and police officer the obligations of the police and with it the legal standard of dangerousness – the law made dangerousness the battlefield, and it has been our Waterloo in American psychiatry.

Why is this the case? Why has the law insisted on this battlefield? I wish to give two answers to this question. The first has to do with the general problem of controlling violence in Western society, and the second has to do with the dilemma of the conflicting moral and empirical grounds for legal policy.

For three decades the American criminal justice system has been staggering; it is now completely overwhelmed by the sheer weight of numbers. This has happened at the same time that our correctional system has completely lost faith in the possibilities of rehabilitation. Our jails and prisons are vastly overcrowded; they have become places of almost uncontrolled violence where inmates daily rape and assault each other. Hobbes's vision of the war of all against all is acted out in what were once euphemistically called reformatories and penitentiaries.

My colleague at Harvard Law School, Professor Dershowitz, argues that this violence in our correctional facilities proves that the legal system is at last working. We are finally confining the "right people." But in a very real sense the criminals have taken over the correctional system in the United States. They determine the nature of the punishment at least as much as the judge and jury. This reality mocks any lofty notion of just retribution or of society imposing the sanctions. Similarly, the great American experiment in juvenile justice is now coming to an end. More and more legal authorities recognize that juveniles cause violent crimes and that the system of *parens patriae* juvenile justice and rehabilitation has, if anything, been counterproductive – a socialization experience in criminality, sadism, and domination. Increasingly, the American Bar Association urges that juveniles be treated as adults: allowed due process and given appropriate punishment.

During the past few years as a spokesman for the American psychiatric establishment, I have learned that journalists, talk show hosts, the educated citizenry, and even some distinguished members of the legal profession believe that somehow psychiatry is responsible for all this. We are attacked as though somehow we had corrupted the criminal justice system. The claims are sometimes inarticulate, but the conviction is passionate and it is growing. Abolition or restriction of the insanity defense is only one example of this claim. A recurrent element in criticism is not only that psychiatric ideas have failed in the area of rehabilitation, but that we also have somehow muddied the moral and behavioral premises that run through the criminal law itself. The most obvious specific example of this loss of moral clarity is the notion of diminished capacity, or more generally the admission of psychiatric testimony on the issue of *mens rea* as well as in support of the insanity defense. Although I believe that these objections have some validity, they are trivial when seen in proper perspective. Forensic psychiatry plays

a very small role in the day-to-day actualities of the criminal justice system. In
a city like New York, for example, very few criminals are apprehended. Some
evade capture throughout their entire criminal careers. A very small percentage
are caught during their first crime. When, if ever, slick first offenders are eventually booked, for, say, an armed robbery, their cases are disposed of by plea
bargaining. First offenders convicted of armed robbery are routinely given suspended sentences. One arrest in a hundred in New York ends in a prison sentence. This state of affairs is not brought about by psychiatry and its supposed
tendency to muddy moral concepts. Psychiatry may be a pimple on the nose of
justice, but the patient has congestive heart failure. If the criminal justice system
has lost some of its ability to deter violence, to protect society, and to exact
retribution, then it needs to look beyond the pimple on its nose.

When one talks to state and federal prosecutors, the real problems of the criminal justice system come into focus. Even if the police did have the capacity to
solve crimes and to arrest criminals, which they do not, it turns out that all too
often the prosecutors lack the resources to try the accused. There are not enough
prosecutors, judges, and juries to try more than a small percentage of those
charged with violent crimes. Ironically, the police increasingly consider the prosecutor to be almost as great a hurdle to law enforcement as the criminal. Many
of the people the police arrest are never charged; charges are dropped, and plea
bargaining is inescapable. The whole system would collapse of its own weight
if every defendant insisted on a trial. Given the limits of prosecutorial resources,
difficult choices have to be made. The favored option is to go after the bad guys,
and one of the most salient features of bad guys is that they are supposedly repeat
violent offenders, dangerous to the public.

When law professors talk about the function of the criminal justice system,
they discourse grandly about retribution, deterrence, rehabilitation, and the protection of society. But when prosecutors talk, it becomes clear that, with limitations of resources, with prisons vastly overcrowded, maximizing the protection
of society has emerged as the only feasible strategy. Prosecutors, of course, have
a political agenda that may complicate this picture, but however this may be,
there is clearly an ongoing effort to target violent offenders, particularly those
who repeat their violent crimes.

This emphasis on dangerousness as the salient variable is not new, of course.
It was central to the sentencing premises of the American Law Institute's Model
Penal Code and the Model Sentencing Act of 1963. It was the central theme in
President Lyndon Johnson's 1967 Commission on Law Enforcement and Administration of Justice. America's National Council on Crime and Delinquency urged
that "the nondangerous offender should not be imprisoned"; instead, the scarce
resources of imprisonment should be reserved for the dangerous offender. Yet at
the same time the president of the council acknowledged that the identification
of dangerous persons remains "the greatest unresolved problem the criminal

justice system faces." Is it not a bizarre system of justice that is prepared to dedicate all of its resources to the confinement of those who cannot be properly identified?

I would like you, the reader, to assume for the moment that the identification of the criminal who will continue to be violent is, in fact, possible. There are now, as there have been in the past, claims that this is possible. The claims come particularly from certain criminologists in Pennsylvania and California. They argue that a small percentage of recidivists are responsible for a disproportionate number of the violent crimes. They urge the prosecutors to focus their resources on these bad guys. To do this, it is necessary to consider such new measures as opening up the records of juvenile offenders. This would entail maximizing the sharing of arrest and conviction criminal records through a centralized computer system, in such a way that it would be possible to learn about an individual's arrest record in every jurisdiction. Assuming that we did all this and the resources of the criminal justice system, police, prosecution, and imprisonment were reserved for these bad guys, what would happen? Before you answer this question, you should also assume the correctness of what the criminologists tell us, which may be different from what many psychiatrists believe – namely, that a convincing argument can be made that violence is not a trait disorder. By acquiring more and more information about violence as a trait disorder we do not add to our knowledge of violent individuals because violence is situational and interactional. We must also assume that street criminals have rational understanding and that they do, in fact, respond to the workings of the criminal justice system. The mugging of tourists in New York City, for example, is highly favored by knowledgeable street criminals because they know that, in the unlikely event that they are caught, the mugged tourists will not return to testify against them and the charges will be dropped. The muggers know how the "muggees" will behave, and they know how the criminal justice system works. The word will go out on the street that "only the bad guys do time." This means that all of the rest of the potential violent criminals (if violence is situational and interactional) have an added inducement to commit crimes that fall just below the line of crimes committed by the "bad guys," and many will go over the line. So depending on the numbers, the justice system itself, by focusing on the dangerous offender, counterproductively might increase violence.

In summary, I have made four points in this section: (a) The criminal justice system is overwhelmed by sheer numbers; (b) the basic strategy of the system is to confine dangerous offenders; (c) it cannot reliably identify dangerous offenders; (d) if it could identify dangerous offenders, there is at least a possibility that the strategy would be counterproductive. In more general terms, I have been discussing the relationship between the mental health and the criminal justice systems.

During the past decade, judges have often criticized the medical model of civil commitment. They have sought to replace it by the criminal justice model. But the real criminal justice model, as I have described it, would hardly seem a useful reform for anything. Moreover, I would suggest that the realities of the criminal justice system are worse than I have depicted them.

The Anglo-American system of justice preaches that it is better for 10 guilty people to go free than for 1 innocent person to be convicted. The reality, however, has little to do with innocent people. The criminal justice system is engaged in triage; it is struggling to make the best use of limited resources in the face of a national disaster. It is this reality that casts a shadow over the mental health system. It is this reality that creates the demand that the mental health system shoulder some of the burden for the protection of society from dangerous individuals.

The criteria of dangerousness

Kant, in the preface to the *Critique of Practical Reason*, wrote that the concept of freedom is "the stumbling block of all empiricists but [it is] the key to the most sublime practical principles to all critical moralists" (Cassirer, 1981, p. 254). I adapt Kant's thoughts to the issue at hand: The concept of dangerousness is the stumbling block of all empirical science, but it is the key to the moral principles adopted recently by judges and legislative bodies critical of psychiatry.

Kant, on the one hand, was making the traditional argument that in a discourse on morality the concept of freedom is essential; without the possibility of freedom, human moral aspiration seems incomprehensible. On the other hand, he was acknowledging that, for those whose work and philosophy were grounded, Kant would say mired, in the empiricism of his day, freedom itself seemed incomprehensible. Kant may or may not have resolved the conflict between these two kinds of discourse. *I have not.* I invoke Kant to emphasize the conflict between the two kinds of discourse. In a discourse of legal rights that are grounded in morality, the concept of dangerousness has emerged as *the* essential element. But in the discourse of contemporary empirical science, dangerousness is demonstrably unworkable. Thus, the *new* law stands with one foot on solid moral ground while the other foot sinks into the empirical quicksand of dangerousness.

It is often said that Kant's ethics are an empty formula for moral conduct, inadequate for deciding concrete individual cases. Similarly, it can be said that dangerousness is an empty formula for legal decisions, inadequate for deciding concrete individual cases.

Let me begin to explain this philosophical rumination by offering the example of capital punishment, which, strangely enough, is relevant to psychiatry in the United States. For many years there has been a legal movement to abolish capital punishment constitutionally as well as legislatively. This movement was inspired not only by moral opposition to capital punishment per se, but also by the apparent pattern of racial discrimination in its application. The data were convincing. Blacks who killed whites were much more apt to be sentenced to death than blacks who killed blacks, or whites who killed whites or blacks. The Supreme Court has resisted abolition of capital punishment, but it has been sensitive to the problem of racial bias. The Court has emphasized that judges and juries ought to be guided in their discretionary decision to impose the death penalty by certain objective criteria. Among those criteria the Court has found that the likelihood of future violence is an acceptable objective standard. Now it seems to me that on a moral basis such a standard is difficult to dispute. If one has to decide which murderers are to be executed, there are strong moral and utilitarian grounds for executing those who pose a continuing threat of violence. If they continue to be violent, it is likely that they feel no remorse and thus deserve a greater punishment.

On utilitarian grounds as well, it makes sense to impose the harshest penalty on those who pose the greatest threat to society. Equally important, if one hopes to avoid bias against racial minorities, the potential for future violence seems to be an objective non-race-related criterion. Thus, in an abstract discourse on the death penalty, future dangerousness seems to have a firm foundation in the legal, constitutional, and moral positions. But this satisfying abstract formula having been adopted, how will it be applied in individual cases? How will the empirical questions of predicting dangerousness be resolved? The answer in some U.S. jurisdictions is that the jury hears testimony from forensic psychiatrists.

Consider the following scenario. The expert witness, relying on his own extensive clinical experience with criminal sociopaths, makes a prediction of dangerousness on behalf of the prosecution. He diagnoses the criminal defendant as a psychopath or sociopath on the basis of his extensive clinical experience with such patients. He asserts that such persons, like the defendant, fail to accept social norms with respect to lawful behavior, lack remorse, and so on. The prognosis, of course, is very bad. Who of us, after all, can promise to cure sociopaths?

Many psychiatrists are convinced of the reliability and validity of the clinical diagnosis of sociopath or, as the *Diagnostic and Statistical Manual of Mental Disorders* (DSM III) (1980) now calls it, antisocial personality disorder. I happen to be a skeptic about this diagnosis for reasons I need not detail here. However, one point must be made: Given the typical life pattern of urban black men, it is safe to say that a significant percentage of them would meet DSM III criteria for antisocial personality, for example, truancy, repeated sexual intercourse in a casual relationship, thefts, vandalism, delinquency before the age of 15, inability to sustain consistent work behavior, failure to plan ahead, conning others, and illegal occupation after 18. By these DSM III criteria, almost all inner-city blacks who come to criminal trial could be diagnosed as antisocial personality. If this thesis is only partly correct, then the diagnosis of antisocial personality, when injected into capital punishment hearings, may restore, under the aegis of clinical psychiatry, the racism that the abstract legal formula was meant to prevent. The empirical application of the legal formula thus defeats the moral objective. The fair standard in theory becomes unfair in practice.

Equally problematic, I believe, is the practice of collapsing predictions of violence into the clinical diagnosis of antisocial personality. Even if we can reliably and validly diagnose antisocial personality disorders and even if many inner-city blacks really have this disorder, there is no evidence that such a diagnosis of *personality disorder* generates valid predictions of violent *behavior*. Furthermore, the whole enterprise of prediction, whether clinical or statistical, is particularly vexed in capital punishment. The defendant, if not executed, will be confined in prison for a lengthy sentence. We all now recognize that clinical prediction of behavior is complicated by the need to take into account the situation in which the person will be. Yet psychiatrists are not asked at the time of capital sentencing to predict the likelihood of violence in prison – that, of course, would be an interesting and difficult question in itself. There is some experience which suggests that violent offenders, particularly multiple murderers, are often model prisoners. Do the courts then mean us to predict whether at some very future time after release the defendant will be dangerous? If so, then they are asking for the kind of long-term predictions that we can assume are particularly unreliable. Finally, if they are asking whether the defendant would be violent if released today, the question is just another legal hypothetical. In answering it, we must speculate about the probability of an impossible event.

The point of all this is to argue that, although the standard of future dangerousness in capital punishment makes sense in legal and moral discourse, and in the abstract is fair, it becomes, in its empirical application to particular cases, unfair. When the Supreme Court of the United States was presented with a legal brief making some of these points and arguing that a Texas death penalty statute with its dangerous standard should be rejected "because it is impossible to predict dangerous behavior," the Court stood its ground and wrote: "It is, of course, not easy to predict future behavior. The fact that such a determination is difficult, however, does not mean that it cannot be made. Indeed, prediction of future criminal conduct is an essential element in many of the decisions rendered throughout our criminal justice system. . . . the task that a Texas jury must perform is thus basically no different from the task performed countless times each day throughout the American system of criminal justice" (*Jurek v. Texas*, 428 U.S. 262, 1976).

All the authoritative scientific statements on clinical and statistical predictions of violence, including recent findings by R. J. Menzies, C. D. Webster, and D. E. Sepejak (chapter 8), say that it cannot be done with any appreciable precision. Yet the Supreme Court with sanguine assurance says that it *is* done every day. It is rather like the man who is asked if he believes in baptism. He answers, "Believe in it? Hell, I've seen it done!" But there is a more subtle lawyer's distinction to be made. The Supreme Court knows that judges and juries have to make many difficult decisions, some of them predictive. These decisions may or may not be correct but, and I quote, "what is essential is that the jury have before it all possible relevant information about the individual defendant whose fate it must determine. Texas law clearly assures that all such evidence will be adduced" (*Jurek*).

To an empiricist, the logic is baffling. Listening to a lot of irrelevant and perhaps false information does not improve one's ability to make predictions. But to the legal mind a decision, even a predictive decision, made in good faith after all the evidence has been weighed, has a kind of procedural validity even if it defies empirical common sense and lacks moral substance. Lawyers may not all agree with this analysis, but it seems to me a fair and not unsympathetic description of the Supreme Court's current posture.

What we have seen, then, in the law is a kind of good-faith prediction that can be defended on procedural grounds even though it lacks empirical justification and moral substance. Whether or not judges believe that this is a rational basis for executing someone, I want to argue that it is not a rational basis for confining someone to a mental hospital.

The relevance of the legal standard of dangerousness to civil commitment

During the past two decades, U.S. courts and legislatures have decided that the medical mode of civil commitment is unconstitutional. Reviewing these developments and concurring in them, one federal judge noted that, along with his concern that personal freedom was at stake, a "close second consideration has been that the diagnosis . . . of mental illness leaves too much to subjective choices by less than neutral individuals."[1] "Less than neutral individuals" refers to psychiatrists. This was the first wave of legal criticism. Psychiatry is too unreliable and too subjective – civil commitment requires an objective legal standard. The objective legal standard is dangerousness.

Once again, I am prepared to recognize the law's struggle to find a fair moral principle to justify the deprivation of liberty. Activists found it in John Stuart Mill, who wrote, "The only purpose for which power can be rightfully exercised over any member of a civilized community against his will is to prevent harm to others" (1961, p. 197).

This was the rationale for the objective standard of civil libertarians. They argued that "dangerous to others" should be the only justification for civil commitment. The sudden popularity of this view among legal authorities was extraordinary. Even under President Nixon and Attorney General Mitchell, I was informed by the Justice Department that in their view dangerousness was constitutionally mandated for civil commitment. When I wrote to the assistant attorney general in charge of the Civil Rights Division, questioning the wisdom and the constitutional necessity of this view, I received a page and a half of irrelevant legal citations – it was a *fait accompli*. It is no longer; even lawyers have come to their senses.

Now it is important to recognize the sense in which dangerousness seemed objective. If one believes that psychiatrists label people crazy just because they espouse different values and different beliefs, then the standard of dangerousness is objective because it protects against the subjective values and standards of psychiatry. This idea of objectivity appeals to Republicans as well as Democrats. But the abstract objective principle is defeated in its application. Once civil libertarians had succeeded in making dangerousness the requisite legal standard, they focused on the inability of psychiatrists to predict dangerousness. Bruce Ennis, then the mental health litigator for the American Civil Liberties Union, wrote with Thomas Litwack, "Psychiatry and the presumption of Expertise: Flipping coins in the Courtroom." My colleague at Harvard Law School, Alan Dershowitz, who had been a major exponent of the objective standard of dangerousness, now reported that psychiatrists were less competent to predict dangerousness than lay people. Suddenly, the legal burden was on psychiatrists to predict dangerousness, and the courts were critical that we could not translate their objective standard into empirical reality.

I emphasize the clash between the two kinds of discourse, moral and empirical. When someone has committed a crime and has been convicted, it may be possible to point to procedures and abstract principles as justifications for punishment. That may be fair in some sense. But when someone is to be confined because he or she is mentally ill, those abstractions cease to be compelling; they are unfair. The decision to be made is not whether it makes sense to confine the alleged patient in a mental hospital. If he or she is not dangerous to others, then the only relevant question is, Will the patient benefit from hospitalization? If the patient is dangerous but has committed no crime, the patient cannot morally be confined on any theory of punishment. What we then confront is the preventive detention decision, and it derives not from jurisprudence but from prudence alone. Prudence depends on empirical reality. Preventive detention decisions may be hedged in by moral principles, but in the end the justification for confining guiltless people is tangible empirical necessity. Psychiatrists can help judges decide whether the patient will benefit from hospitalization, but they cannot help judges with the long-term prediction of dangerousness. Nor, I would claim, can judges make these predictions on their own procedural grounds and justify them.

The dilemma is unresolvable; the objective legal standard is unworkable because no empirical standards exist. The fact that we may be able to make short-term predictions of violence only adds to our problem. If we use such short-term predictions as a basis for confining people, then how do we decide whether it is safe to discharge them? This is the most pressing clinical problem in psychiatry today. How do we decide when to release someone whose initial confinement was based on a short-term prediction of dangerousness? Recently, a group of us were asked to consult with the Secret Service personnel who are charged with protecting the president. In the course of that consultation, we learned that one of the chief problems confronting the Secret Service is deciding when it is safe to remove a person from their files once that person has been identified as a threat to the president. They have the same problem that we do, and their files keep expanding. Years ago, our solution was the same: We "warehoused" these people. The law no longer allows this, and furthermore the mental helath system is now dominated by a philosophy based on short-term confinement. The better the quality of psychiatric care, the greater is the pressure to restore patients to treatment programs in the community.

As more and more dangerous patients are processed through a system of short-term confinement, there will be more instances of violence by former mental patients, and there will be more of the second-generation criticism of the psychiatric profession – "You are not protecting the public." That is why the attorney general's Task Force on Violent Crimes appointed by President Reagan recognized these developments and suggested that statutes be passed to allow the victims of violence by former prisoners to bring civil lawsuits for damages against those making the release decisions. These lawsuits, the task force suggested, would increase the care with which discharge decisions are made. Now I favor compensation for victims, but it is absurd, in light of what we know, to think that threats of lawsuits will lead to better predictions when there are no solid empirical grounds on which to make those predictions.

The morality of law and its jurisprudence is based on a theory of acts that have been committed. Nowhere is there a coherent jurisprudence of preventive detention. If there were such a jurisprudence, it would have to be based on empirical studies. Such studies do not now exist. Psychiatrists and others who appear in court to offer predictions of violence allow the courts to continue to deny that they have one foot in quicksand. This, in the long run, is a disservice to the law and to the attempts to establish psychiatry and psychology as scientific disciplines.

Note

1 See Judge King in *Suzuki v. Quisenberry*, A1 F. Supp. 1113, 1135 (D.C. Hawaii 1976).

References

Cassirer, E. *Kant's life and thought*. New Haven: Yale University Press, 1981.

Diagnostic and statistical manual of mental disorders (3rd ed.). Washington, D.C.: American Psychiatric Association, 1980.

Ennis, B. J., & Litwack, T. R. Psychiatry and the presumption of expertise: Flipping coins in the courtroom. *California Law Review*, 1974, *62*, 693–752.

Mill, J. S. On liberty. In M. Cohen (Ed.), *The philosophy of John Stuart Mill*. New York: Modern Library, 1961.

Stone, A. A. *Mental health and the law: A system in transition*. New York: Aronson, 1976.

Stone, A. A. The right to refuse treatment. *Archives of General Psychiatry*, 1981, *38*, 358–62.

2   Dangerousness, mental disorder, and politics

Cyril Greenland

Although more than 90% of all the articles and books ever written on this topic have probably been published in the past 20 years, the association between violence and mental disorders has been recognized since ancient times. In drawing attention to this historical fact, I suggest that problems of this type, which have plagued humankind since the dawn of history, are unlikely to be solved by semasiological juggling or by modern technology. Because technology is never value free or without cost, at best it can succeed only in transforming or redistributing rather than eradicating the symptoms of human distress.

It is also necessary to emphasize that, despite the lively and sometimes illuminating criticisms of psychiatry by writers such as Foucault (1978), Szasz (1968), Kittrie (1971), and many others, mental illness continues to be a reality and that throughout history, in all cultures, special arrangements have been made to deal with mentally ill offenders. For example, the notion that victims of mental illness should not be regarded as fully responsible for their crimes was clearly established in ancient Greek and in early Jewish and Roman laws. Long before psychiatry as we know it evolved, other public officials were entrusted with the task of determining whether a mad person was responsible for his or her criminal acts and, if so, when and under what circumstances he or she could be safely restored to society.

The thirteenth-century case of Richard of Cheddestan (Walker, 1968, pp. 20–3), also known as Richard Blofot, indicates that a legal procedure similar to the Canadian lieutenant governor's warrant was used in England as early as 1270. It seems that Richard Blofot, in a state of frenzy, killed his wife and children. Having been found not guilty by reason of insanity, he was held in prison for 6 years. Acting on orders from Edward I, a group of officials, including the sheriff of Norfolk, examined Richard Blofot and reported, "The same Richard is well enough; but it cannot safely be said that he is so restored to soundness of mind that there would not be danger in setting him free, especially when the heat of summer is increasing, lest worse befall" (p. 23). With some minor modifications the equivalent of this statement might well be part of a report prepared by the

25

advisory review board that is responsible for reviewing the status of patients detained in Ontario under a lieutenant governor's warrant.

This case example serves two purposes. It supports my contention that the assessment of dangerousness, on behalf of the state, has a long history. It also serves to introduce Dr. Szasz's (1968, pp. 144–5) argument that psychiatrists wrongly diagnose mental illness in people who engage in destructive behavior. He writes, "There is no evidence that mental patients are a greater source of danger to society than nonmental patients," and "The myth of the 'dangerous mental patient' dies hard" (p. 144).

The case of Valentine Shortis provides a dramatic example of the situation that Szasz quite properly condemns. The essential details of this case (Greenland, 1962) are as follows. In 1894, 20-year-old Valentine Shortis, a "remittance man" from Ireland living in Valleyfield, Quebec, without any apparent motive or malice, shot and killed some of his workmates. Dr. C. K. Clarke, one of Canada's leading psychiatrists who was called by the defense, reported, "Shortis is an imbecile and suffers from homicidal mania" (p. 262). Clarke concluded, "To the alienist the case does not present many difficulties and no doubt when the family history is supplied a flood of light will be thrown on the matter as cases of insanity of this type (moral imbecile with homicidal mania, paranoid class) have a genealogy that supplies a satisfactory reason for the degeneracy made so apparent by a crime of this atrocious order" (p. 262).

Similar evidence was provided for the defense by other leading psychiatrists, including Dr. Daniel Clark and Dr. R. M. Bucke. As a result, Shortis was found not guilty by reason of insanity and confined to the Kingston Penitentiary. Eleven years later Dr. C. K. Clarke visited Kingston Penitentiary and examined Shortis. The following is an extract from his report. "A more typical specimen of the paranoid dement could not be found. . . . Whatever impression may have existed in some minds regarding his mental disease at the time of his trial, there can no longer be any doubt on the part of the most skeptical" (p. 264). Clarke also noted, "A marked facial tremor, particularly on the left side; the tongue when protruded had a coarse tremor and so had the extended hands. Articulation was defective and the voice manneristic. He spoke with a marked French accent. Ideas of persecution were also noted." Clarke's diagnosis was "Valentine Shortis – Paranoia, Incurable" (p. 264).

Dr. Clarke's untimely death in 1924 prevented him from following up this case. But, contrary to his clinical prediction, Shortis did not deteriorate in prison. Instead, like violins and good wine, he improved enormously with age. After 42 years of incarceration at the age of 62, Shortis was released into the community under the care of police detective John Kearney. When I interviewed him in 1961, Mr. Kearney told me that Shortis was a familiar figure in Toronto. He attracted attention because of his unusual dress, beard, and monocle. He spent a great deal of time recruiting for the Toronto regiments and used to stop young men and tell them that "Hitler had to be beaten or they would live in slavery" (p. 267).

Shortis died in 1941. Because there was no postmortem examination of his brain, it is difficult to confirm or reject Dr. Clarke's pessimistic diagnosis. All that remains as evidence of Shortis's personality is the obituary submitted to the press by the deputy provincial secretary, C. F. Neeland: "I had Shortis under my care for 15 years when I was Reformatory Superintendant. During those years I always found he took a stand for good law and order. He gave sound advice to hundreds of young prisoners and was a good influence with them. As a result a lot of young prisoners have to thank him to-day that they are now good citizens" (p. 267). So much for the diagnosis of "moral imbecility."

The Shortis case illustrates that psychiatry, no less than other professional disciplines, operates in a given political, historical, and cultural context. The notion of professional independence and freedom from political influence is, of course, a dangerous delusion. This matter will be considered later in a somewhat different context.

The remainder of this chapter is organized under three headings: (a) the politics of dangerousness, (b) the limits of clinical prediction, and (c) alternative strategies. The third and concluding section is based mainly on my own rather eccentric contributions to research over the past dozen or so years.

The politics of dangerousness

It is obvious that the expression "violent and dangerous" in the context of mental disorder represents a sociopolitical judgment rather than a psychiatric diagnosis. Because violence and aggression are promoted rather than condemned in our society, the tendency to behave violently in violence-prone situations cannot be regarded as necessarily abnormal. Thus, without a precise knowledge of the situation in which violence is used, it is often impossible to determine the extent to which the violence is specifically related to mental illness rather than to the social situation. A tragic example of this is the recently reported destruction of unwanted female infants in China.

Because it is frequently mentioned in other texts (e.g., Monahan, 1981) it is unnecessary to elaborate the arbitrary decision to be concerned about violence related to mental illness while ignoring, for example, carnage on the highways, the dreadful consequences of environmental pollution, and the omnipresent threat of a nuclear holocaust. It is necessary, however, to comment on another form of dangerous behavior that seems to be increasing in our war-torn world. I refer to political terrorism and the incarceration and torture of so-called political dissidents. Beginning, perhaps, with Herod in his "massacre of the innocents," totalitarian governments have engaged in what M. Falcoff (quoted by Walzer, 1981) describes as the "abolition of innocence."

"This pre-requisite of a successful reign of terror," writes Falcoff, "is always accompanied by multiplications not so much of a suspicious person as of a whole category of suspects." In revolutionary China and the USSR, bourgeois intellectual revisionists and capitalistic reactionaries are regarded as dangerous enemies of the state. In Argentina, "liberal journalists" and social scientists, including psychoanalysts, have been defined as dangerous, imprisoned without trial, and tortured to death. In Canada, until recently, the mentally retarded were regarded as a major social menace (Greenland, 1963).

The *état dangereux* idea has a long history in criminology. Concerned about the high rate of crime and the general state of lawlessness in France in the 1830s, the Academie des Sciences Morales et Politiques arranged an essay competition. The subject of the essay was as follows. "Based on positive observation, study the elements which, in Paris or any other major city, constitute the segment of the population considered dangerous because of its vice, lack of education and miserable living conditions, and indicate means by which government, the leisured classes and intelligent, diligent workers could improve this dangerous and depraved class" (quoted in Fregier, 1977).

The competition was won by H. A. Fregier, a chief of police. In 1840 he published a two-volume work entitled *Des Classes Dangereuses dans les Grandes Villes*. This title is somewhat misleading because Fregier identifies two groups of dangerous people. There are violent and aggressive criminals and those who, without committing any crime, pose a more direct and serious threat to the moral structure of society. Fregier observes that what both groups have in common is poverty, which, he says, is a direct result of their evil ways. His conclusion was: "Danger to society grows and becomes increasingly serious as the conditions of the poor deteriorate through vice and, more serious still, through laziness. When a poor man who is exposed to bad habits ceases to work, he becomes a public enemy because he ignores the supreme law of work" (vol. 1, p. 7).

The Lombrosian concept that certain individuals have a psychobiological disposition to commit crimes was recognized and endorsed by legislators in Britain. The habitual offender legislation, part of the Prevention of Crime Act, was introduced in England and Wales in 1908. The basic idea, which would have pleased Fregier, was not to punish a person for his or her crime, but to protect society by removing the incorrigible offender from its midst.

Despite the growing evidence that it had proved to be a conspicuous and notorious failure in Britain, preventive detention was introduced into Canadian legislation in 1947. The role to be played by psychiatrists in relation to the criminal sexual psychopath legislation, introduced in the following year, was clearly and perhaps cynically articulated by the minister of justice, the Honorable James

Lorimer Ilsley. In response to a question from Mr. John Diefenbaker, the member from Prince Albert, concerning the role of the provincial attorneys general, the minister of justice replied:

The consequences being so serious so far as the deprivation of liberty is concerned, it was felt that the Attorney General, who is responsible for the maintenance of order and the enforcement of law in the province, should consent to action against the person in that way and to the nomination of these psychiatrists, one nominated by the Minister of Justice, with a view to getting a finding that might land the accused in custody for a great many years.[1]

In other words, he believed that expert psychiatric testimony in the courtroom regarding the dangerousness and treatability of the offender was necessary to secure lengthy prison sentences.

The accuracy of the honorable minister's assessment and the willingness of some Canadian psychiatrists to be used in this disreputable legal process has been fully documented in several studies (Greenland, 1977, 1984; Price and Gold, 1976) on which I have been privileged to work. This research confirms that with the complicity of a few psychiatrists the least dangerous sexual offenders, most of them homosexual pedophiles, tend on the whole to be incarcerated for much longer periods than their truly dangerous counterparts, including violent heterosexual rapists. The intrusion of politics into the clinical assessment of dangerousness is painfully evident in the extremely punitive attitude of our government toward homosexuals and the use of psychiatry as an instrument of repression.

The limits of clinical prediction

It should be obvious by now that the clinical prediction of dangerousness is a difficult and unenviable task. Overprediction results in the unnecessary use of compulsion, such as prolonged indeterminate imprisonment or involuntary hospitalization in a maximum-security facility. Underprediction may result in suicide, homicide, or serious assaults on innocent victims. Most clinicians who have a professional and legal duty to make such decisions are aware of these agonizing dilemmas. Statistical studies of the prediction of dangerousness among discharged mental patients indicate a high rate of error, usually in the direction of overprediction. Until recently, relatively little attention has been paid to the havoc caused by the "false negatives." These are the people who kill or maim others after being considered safe for discharge. Monahan (1981), whose own thinking on these matters has turned full circle over the past 5 years, now seeks a balance between "the patient's right not to be a false positive and the victim's right not to be set upon by a false negative" (p. 169).

My early research on the work of the special security hospitals in England and Wales (Greenland, 1969, 1970a, 1970b) confirmed that psychiatrists and the judiciary tended to overestimate the risks of violence and dangerous behavior among mentally ill offenders. This is the basis of the argument that psychiatrists are responsible for restraining three or four patients in order to prevent one from committing another violent offense. In a playful mood, Dr. Barry Boyd, formerly medical director of the maximum-security hospital of Penetanguishene, Ontario, said he believed that only 10% of the patients detained under his care would kill again on discharge. He would be delighted, he said, to set the remaining 90% free if someone could tell him reliably who they were. Although not meant to be taken seriously, this pragmatic approach to the problem of prediction places a high value on protecting the public from further harm. The approach taken by the critics of psychiatry is, by contrast, academic and speculative. They assume the role of a person observing a poker game.

He sees all the hands and knows which cards are being dealt. He even knows which cards are still in the deck. Armed with this information, he also knows exactly how the hand should be played and the game won. However, if he were a player rather than an observer, making rapid decisions in the heat of the moment, his level of competence would inevitably decline. Without stretching the analogy too far, I want to suggest that the clinician in his day-to-day work is in a similar position. Access to all information as if he were an observer would obviously enable him to make better decisions. But unlike the critics, psychiatrists rarely enjoy the luxury of academic detachment and prescience.[2]

It is not surprising that the language employed by the critics of psychiatry in the debate over the prediction of dangerousness has an evangelic or even a messianic fervor. For example, in an otherwise valuable paper, Cocozza and Steadman (1976) conclude: "The data just presented constitute the most definitive evidence available on the lack of expertise and accuracy of psychiatric predictions of dangerousness. The findings of this study taken together with the other works reviewed in this paper, would appear to present clear and convincing evidence of the inability of psychiatrists or anyone else to predict dangerousness accurately" (p. 1099). Then, as if to confirm their rhetorical claim, Cocozza and Steadman conclude with this challenge: "Although we have suggested that the question is not yet answered conclusively, it would appear that there is enough evidence on the inadequacy of such predictions to now place the burden of proof on psychiatrists and others to demonstrate that dangerousness can be accurately predicted" (p. 1101).

Operation Baxtrom, which resulted in the release of 969 "insane criminals" (*Baxtrom v. Herold,* 383 US. 107, 1966) provided Cocozza and Steadman (1976) with what they regarded as incontrovertible evidence of psychiatric incompetence. These otherwise brilliant critics, however, overlooked the fact that very few, if any, of the physicians employed in the Matteawan or Dannemora State Hospitals were professionally qualified or board-certified psychiatrists. This was also true in the notorious Donaldson (1976) case (*O'Connor v. Donaldson,* USSC,

1975). The key defendants were not psychiatrists. The medical superintendant, legally responsible for Donaldson's 15 years of confinement, was medically qualified as a gynecologist.

Although they misjudged the lack of psychiatric competence, the studies by Cocozza and Steadman provide valuable but depressing information about slovenly administrative and diagnostic procedures employed in New York State in the 1970s. Commenting on this, the English Floud committee (Floud & Young, 1981) stated that the studies just referred to ''provide better evidence of bad practice than of the state of the art of assessing dangerousness; their findings bear more on the practice than the theoretical problems of ensuring just predictive judgements'' (p. 30).

Preoccupied with the need to demonstrate the incompetence of psychiatry, most of the critics have been reluctant to examine the practical alternatives to the current methods of clinical assessment. Megargee (1981), a highly respected researcher, admits that ''the first methodological problem in the study of predicting dangerous behavior is that there is no systematic scientific way to test our predictions'' (p. 180). But even if it were possible to do, the excessive number of ''false positives'' would still be a problem. This issue was considered in a Rand Corporation study of ''violent predators.'' The authors, Chaiken and Chaiken (1982), confirmed ''that it would be extremely difficult to develop, at this time, a statistical model that could be fairly used by the courts to identify and incarcerate for longer periods'' (p. 8).

My aim in presenting this information is neither to score debating points against Steadman and his colleagues, nor to defend psychiatry. But I hope to show that, once a person has been found guilty, or not guilty by reason of insanity, of a serious offense involving violence, the issue of actuarial prediction of a tendency to repeat the offense is of little consequence in the initial decision regarding the disposition of the offender. This becomes an issue only when the patient or the prisoner has to be considered for release or for parole. This difficult task, which should involve both statistical and clinical prediction, must be approached with concern for the rights of the public as well as the offender. Above all, we need a sense of professional modesty, which is often lacking in the polarized literature on this topic. It is comforting to know, however, that over the years the protagonists are becoming less belligerent and much more open to constructive criticism. For example, in his introduction to *Predicting Violent Behavior,* Monahan (1981) confesses that at several points in its gestation, his book had different subtitles. He writes, ''When I was beginning the monograph the working subtitle was 'Why You Can't Do It' '' (p. 19). About halfway through he changed the subtitle to ''How to Do It and Why You Shouldn't.'' By the time the book was finished, he was toying with a new subtitle: ''How to Do It and When to Do It.''

On a more serious note, Monahan points out the development of his thinking about the clinical prediction of dangerousness as it moved through the following sequences: "from an empirical distaste for the task, to an ethical aversion to engaging in it, to reluctant concession that there may be circumstances in which the prediction of dangerousness is both empirically possible and ethically appropriate" (p. 19).

Monahan's pragmatic approach echoes the conclusions of the Canadian Committee on Corrections (1969), which, in supporting indeterminate sentencing, recommended that the assessment of dangerousness be undertaken in special psychiatric centers to be built and administered by the Canadian Penitentiary Services. The Ouimet committee's recommendations resulted in the passage of the Serious Personal Injury Offence (Canadian Criminal Code, part 21) in 1977, which replaced the dangerous sexual offender legislation. Unfortunately, the Ouimet committee failed to anticipate that Canadian courts would broaden the definition of dangerousness. In a recent case (*Queen v. Milne*, Provincial Court of British Columbia, 1980), the Crown coopted a psychiatrist to testify that, although the offender, a homosexual pedophile, was not dangerous, he was nevertheless an evil person.

The Floud committee (Floud & Young, 1981) in the United Kingdom, which also recommended the use of indeterminate sentences, hoped that it would be reserved by statute for offenders who cause grave harm or death or who commit serious sexual assaults, and so on. But the Canadian experience, referred to earlier, suggests that British courts, aided perhaps by psychiatric experts, might also apply indeterminate sentences to offenders whose behavior is socially repugnant rather than dangerous. Although this fear was not actually expressed, the Floud committee recommended that psychiatrists who are required to report on dangerous offenders be carefully selected by the courts to ensure that they are well qualified for the task.

Despite all the criticism directed against it in the United Kingdom, the United States, and Canada, it seems that indeterminate or protective sentences are here to stay. This means that in the absence of publicly acceptable alternatives psychiatrists will continue to be called on by the courts to predict dangerousness or by parole boards or advisory review boards to determine if and when a dangerous offender or patient is fit to be returned to the community. So, until more humane and effective methods are developed and sanctioned by society, psychiatrists should stop being apologetic and defensive and strive to improve their skills in this difficult and contentious area. Because we must also conclude that the actuarial or purely clinical or diagnostic approaches to the prediction of dangerousness are ineffective as well as socially unacceptable, some alternative strategies are considered in the final section of these reflections.

Alternative strategies

Earlier in the chapter I referred to my research on the function and operation of the three special hospitals in England (Greenland, 1969, 1970a, 1970b). This work evolved from my study of the operation of the mental health tribunals (Greenland, 1970c). In the course of this research I was privileged not only to read all the relevant legal and clinical records, but also to interview the patients, their relatives, psychiatrists, and nurses and finally to sit in on the hearings where the decisions were taken to retain the patients or to order their release. Because the patients had already demonstrated a capacity for violence, the hearings concerned with the special hospitals patients were of particular interest to me.

Functioning albeit as a visiting anthropologist, my primary interest was in the systems, rituals, and outcomes of decision making rather than in the strictly clinical and legal issues. From this perspective it soon became clear that only in rare and usually very obvious cases were psychiatrists adamantly opposed to the patient's release. Instead of being considered the final arbiter in the decision to retain or release difficult patients, tribunals were not infrequently used either to test the patient's readiness or as a vehicle for sharing responsibility when perplexing decisions had to be taken.

In reaching decisions, tribunals are required to examine all the circumstances surrounding the patient's admission to hospitals, his or her family situation, skills, work records, previous hospital admissions or offenses, relationship to the victim, response to treatment, behavior in hospital, and so on. This broad assessment enabled the tribunal to reach a high degree of consensus about the patient's fitness for discharge. Although mistakes were made and some patients had to be readmitted, except for several suicides there was a very low incidence of criminal assault.

At unanticipated outcome of the tribunal's mode of inquiry was that the initial offense, which resulted in the patient being found not guilty by reason of insanity or unfit to stand trial, was considered in its broadest social context rather than in the context of the mental illness. For example, in the case of a very depressed and socially isolated woman who killed her children, the inquiry revealed that after abortive attempts to seek help the patient decided that suicide was the only solution. To save her children from further suffering the mother fed them tranquilizers provided by her family physician and then drowned them in the bath. After taking an overdose of tranquilizers herself, cutting her wrists, and turning ᴏn the gas she called the police, who arrived in time to save her life. There was no doubt that the patient was not, in the usual sense, a dangerous person. The psychiatrist, who admitted that the patient had made an excellent recovery from her severe depression, was concerned that on discharge from hospital she might kill herself. After ascertaining that she had excellent family support and good job prospects, the tribunal decided that because the patient no longer required hospitalization and would not benefit from it she should be discharged, provided that adequate aftercare arrangements were made for her. Follow-up a year later showed that, after some initial difficulty, requiring a brief admission to a local hospital, the patient was self-supporting and managing very well on her own.

This case and many others with similar backgrounds and outcomes prompted the development of my program of research on violence and dangerous behavior, which I started at the Clarke Institute of Psychiatry in the Section on Social Pathology directed by Hans Mohr. Dr. Mohr had already established an international reputation for his work on pedophilia and exhibitionism (Mohr, Turner, and Jerry, 1964) and on matricide and mental illness (McKnight et al., 1966). Very much like my own, his research approach was phenomenological. The objectives were practical and strictly empirical. We were not guided by any specific theoretical system, nor were we concerned to discover causes or explanations for the offenses, but we did attempt to learn everything we could about the offense, the offender, the victim(s), and the history and consequences of the phenomenon as a whole. This approach, borrowed from Mohr, has influenced almost all of my research. I will mention three pieces of work that support the need for an alternative approach to the problem of identifying and managing violent and dangerous people.

Referring to the notorious Whitman case, Ralph Banay (1967) a distinguished forensic psychiatrist, wrote: "The question raised by impulsive murder, including multiple homicide, is no longer, Why did he do it? but Why wasn't it prevented? Although each case presents a unique combination of environmental and pathological factors, the underlying elements are so repetitively familiar that there need be no mystery about the mechanisms of the murderous outbursts" (p. 1). The challenging suggestion that people who kill often signal their intentions but fail to elicit the necessary help or restraint is one of the most useful leads in evaluating and, it is to be hoped, preventing dangerous behavior. Support for this view came from our Violent Offences against Persons Study (Greenland, 1972). This was a study of 91 patients detained in Ontario hospitals under lieutenant governor's warrants (LGWs). All of them, 69 men and 22 women, had committed violent offenses, including 70 homicides, involving 50 men and 20 women. A comparable study was made of a random, one in four, sample of male penitentiary inmates matched for offenses. The poor quality of data available from this cohort limited the value of the comparison. There was, however, a substantial overlap between the men in both cohorts. Half of the LGWs had a previous history of psychiatric treatment. The same proportion had previous convictions. One-third of them involved violent offenses. A similar proportion of male inmates had previous convictions. One-third of them also had previous, that is, before the current offense, admissions to mental hospitals.

Striking differences were observed between the male and female LGWs. Almost exclusively, the women killed or attempted to kill family members. Children and husbands were the major victims. Almost half of the women had a history of depression, for which they had been treated. About half of the men, 47%, killed strangers. This suggests that homicide committed by women is phenomenologically quite different from the same act committed by men.

Because this has been described elsewhere (Greenland, 1980a), I shall mention only briefly the typology of violent offenders that emerged from this study. Although still very crude, it may have some heuristic if not predictive value.

1. *Chronic antisocial* (LGWs, 35%; penitentiary inmates, 60%). These men are habitually aggressive. Their behavior in the form of assaultiveness combined with alcoholism suggests chronic social maladaptation. Megargee's term, "undercontrolled," applies to most of them.
2. *Psychotic episode* (LGWs, 56%; penitentiary inmates, 36%). The violence is usually associated with an acute psychotic episode with a marked delusional system and/or a loss of contact with reality. The offense is frequently associated with a buildup of problems and unbearable emotional tension, which is relieved by the assault. Some of these offenders expressed the feeling of being locked in an unbearable situation, described by McKnight et al. (1966) in their matricide study.
3. *Episodic and situational violence* (LGWs, 6%; penitentiary inmates, 4%). This type of violence is usually the result of recurrent manic–depressive illness, organic brain dysfunction, or cyclical alcoholism, resulting in rage states. Similar cases have been described by Mark and Ervin (1970) and by Williams (1969).
4. *Extended suicide* (LGWs, 21%; penitentiary inmates, nil). There were 1 man and 20 women in this LGW group. They killed for altruistic reasons as a form of extended suicide. Previously diagnosed and treated clinical depression was common. Help-seeking and warning behavior was most frequently observed in this group.

It is important to emphasize that "help seeking" usually consists of unequivocal appeals to physicians, social workers, or the police for immediate assistance or restraint. Warning signals, best recognized by hindsight, consist of overt or veiled threats combined with abnormal or disturbing behavior that should have alerted the victim(s) and/or others to take evasive or defensive action. Such prodromal events were clearly demonstrated in the unpublished study by Greenland and Rosenblatt (1975) of murder followed by suicide in Ontario during the period from 1966 to 1970. At least nine (19%) of the murder–suicide offenders had made previous suicide attempts.

Further evidence of help-seeking behavior comes from my research on child abuse deaths (Greenland, 1980b). The majority of children who die as a result of abuse or neglect are already known to child welfare agencies. This finding is supported by other studies. Scott (1973), in his study of 29 fatal battered baby cases, reported that three-quarters of the male assailants gave unmistakable warning of their subsequent actions. In an earlier paper from Glasgow, Bennie and Sclare (1969) concluded, on the basis of their case studies, that "five of the ten patients had seen a doctor immediately preceding the crime, in some cases to complain about the child's behavior and to seek help in management" (p. 978).

These authors ask if a higher degree of medical awareness might have prevented some of these tragedies. What should this awareness consist of? In addition to recognizing and responding appropriately to help-seeking or warning behavior, clinicians must increase their sense of confidence about discussing murderous feelings with their patients or clients. The impulse to prescribe tranquilizers for anxious and depressed mothers of young children should be strenuously resisted. It is also vital for the clinician to remember that the impulse to kill is almost invariably episodic and victim specific. Chapman (1959), in a valuable study of obsessions of infanticide, pointed out that many of his patients were extremely fearful of incipient insanity and the loss of control. This fear, I have discovered, also appears prodromally in other forms of interpersonal violence. An exploration of the operation of the patient's inner and outer control against his or her murderous impulses is vitally important in the identification and management of high-risk cases.

The fact that impulse control is substantially reduced by alcohol is well known. In my own research (Greenland, 1980a) alcohol was a factor in more than half of the homicide cases. In one-third of these cases both the victims and assailants were intoxicated. Many sex offenders also claim to have been drunk when the offense was committed. The same is true of wife abusers. Fortunately, for most of us alcohol produces a state of euphoria, relaxation, and the illusion of happiness, but for a limited number of tipplers, the ingestion of a small quantity of alcohol results in paradoxical rage reactions. In vulnerable individuals, alcohol combined with one of the benzodiazepines may sometimes trigger rage states. Another use of alcohol, not to my knowledge mentioned in the literature, is that of self-incapacitation. Several sadistic sex murderers in our series used alcohol for this purpose for many years. Periodic binges, enabling the offender to become stuporous for several days, served to obliterate compulsive sexual fantasies involving killing and mutilating the victims – often children. Some of these men also incapacitated themselves by attacking police officers in order to be arrested or by getting drunk and walking into traffic, hoping to be killed or at least seriously injured.

These observations, which came from careful listening rather than talking to dangerous offenders or reading about them in case records, prompted me to formulate what, with uncharacteristic modesty, I have called Greenland's rule:

The urge to kill or seriously harm another person is almost invariably accompanied by an equal but opposite urge to be restrained from killing or harming. Although enormously important in the clinical assessment of violence, this rule is impossible to prove except in retrospect. However, our data on several hundred serious offenses, including homicide, rape, murder–suicide, arson, and child abuse, confirm that in at least half of the cases in which the information was available, the offender was being seen by a psychiatrist, physician, social worker, or probation officer, or some combination of helpers, immediately before the tragedy.

I assume that the old-fashioned practice of taking a comprehensive social history might have enabled at least some of these patients to reveal and the clinician to understand their attempts to seek help and regain control over destructive impulses. The modern practice of "crisis intervention," which treats human problems as discrete and ahistorical events, effectively prevents us from seeing the person and his or her problem in a more complete or holistic fashion. It also exempts us from the burden of fully understanding or caring for that person in anything but a fragmented fashion. Perhaps this explains our reluctance to observe warning signals and respond effectively to help-seeking behaviors.

In concluding this chapter, I will present and comment on four findings from my own research and reading about the phenomenology of criminal violence. I hope that this will contribute to our understanding of assessment.

1. The urge to kill is episodic in nature and never a permanent state. With rare exceptions, individuals are never dangerous all the time.
2. Dangerous behavior is usually an age-, sex-, victim-, and situation-specific activity.
3. The offenders are usually young, poor, and ill-educated men.
4. The victims are usually women or children.

These findings tend to be ignored or discounted by clinicians who favor actuarial or psychodiagnostic approaches to the assessment of dangerousness. Statistical and diagnostic procedures provide a semblance of science, which, by the process of mystification, renders the exercise professionally respectable. This enables us to avoid coming to terms with what McGrath (1982) calls the "ambient circumstances of the offence which gave a presumption of danger in the first place" (p. 95). He asks us to consider: "What were the triggers and what were the provocations? What were the controls or lack of controls?" (p. 95).

Other forensic experts and researchers, including Megargee (1981), Monahan (1981), Quinsey (1979), and Steadman (1981), in their later publications, have also begun to emphasize the situational or contextual aspects of dangerousness. Further progress will depend, however, on the ability of psychiatrists to accept the offender fully as a person and recognize the connections between his or her murderous impulses and the experience of economic, political, and psychological powerlessness. Although most physicians recognize the close relationship between poverty, powerlessness, and disease, the impact of this association on the practice of medicine has been very modest. This is especially so in forensic psychiatry, which still acts as if the impulse to rape, maim, or kill resides like malignancy within the individual offender. The fact that electroencephalographic abnormalities are often found in this population is, in the larger context, of little consequence. A high incidence of head injuries and neuropathy caused by lead and other highly toxic environmental contaminants is also correlated with poverty.

Short of a social revolution, what are the alternatives? There are two basic options. The first involves incapacitating an increasing number of dangerous offenders by incarcerating them for long periods in maximum-security prisons. The other, which recognizes the baleful consequences of poverty and social deprivation, involves the mutual sharing of power, information, and experience among hospital or prison administrators, clinicians and researchers, and patients or offenders.

Starting on a modest scale, I propose the establishment of special research units planned and managed by selected inmates in maximum- or medium-security prisons. Responsible to independent advisory boards with some university affiliation, the inmates should be given access to training, facilities, research funds, consultants, and a clear mandate to explore the phenomenology of criminal violence and its prevention. One of the first projects could be the establishment of an experimental debriefing unit for rapists or multiple murderers such as Clifford Olsen (Ferry & Inwood, 1982).

Coming back to earth, we must recognize that, although there is a desperate need for innovative ideas, the chances of persuading the authorities to adopt them is remote. This is because changes that upset existing power relationships threaten the economic and political structures in which penology and psychiatry thrive. However, the widespread increase in malignant violence, an inevitable consequence of social and political inequality, magnified by the imminent threat of nuclear disaster, compels us to make difficult choices. We can opt for peace and social justice, which involves the planned sharing of power and resources, or we can define the underprivileged members of society as social enemies and control them, as instruments of political repression, by the use of long-term incarceration, psychopharmacology, or neurosurgery. Because the traditional shelter of academic and professional neutrality is now part of the battlefield, there is no escape from these painful dilemmas.

Notes

1 5 H.C. Deb. 5195–200, 5203 at 5197 (1948).
2 I have lost the source of this invaluable quotation.

References

Banay, R. S. Point of view: Multiple homicide – A neglected peril. *Corrective Psychiatry and Journal of Social Therapy,* 1967, *13,* 1–4.

Bennie, E. H., & Sclare, A. B. The battered child syndrome. *American Journal of Psychiatry,* 1969, *125,* 975–9.

Canadian Committee on Corrections (Ouimet Committee) report. Ottawa: Queen's Printer, 1969.

Chaiken, J. M., & Chaiken, M. R. Varieties of criminal behavior: Summary and policy implications. *Bulletin of the Canadian Association for the Prevention of Crime,* 1982, *3,* 8.

Chapman, A. K. Obsessions of infanticide. *Archives of General Psychiatry,* 1959, *1,* 12–16.

Cocozza, J. J., & Steadman, H. J. The failure of psychiatric prediction of dangerousness: Clear and convincing evidence. *Rutgers Law Review,* 1976, *29,* 1048–1101.

Donaldson, K. *Insanity inside out.* New York: Crown, 1976.

Ferry, J., & Inwood, D. *The Olsen murders.* Vancouver: Cameo Books, 1982.

Floud, J., & Young, W. *Dangerousness and criminal justice* (Howard League for Penal Reform). London: Heinemann, 1981.

Foucault, M. About the concept of the "dangerous individual" in 19th century legal psychiatry. In D. N. Weisstub (Ed.), *Law and psychiatry: Proceedings of an international symposium.* New York: Pergamon, 1978.

Fregier, H. A. *Des classes dangereuses dans les grandes villes.* Geneva: Slatkine-Megariotis Reprints, 1977. (Originally published, Paris: 1840.)

Greenland, C. L'Affaire Shortis and the Valleyfield murders. *Canadian Psychiatric Association Journal,* 1962, *7,* 261–71.

Greenland, C. The treatment of the mentally retarded in Ontario: A historical note. *Canadian Psychiatric Association Journal,* 1963, *8,* 328–36.

Greenland, C. The three special hospitals in England and patients with dangerous, violent or criminal propensities. *Medicine, Science and the Law.* 1969, *9*(4), 253–65.

Greenland, C. The three special hospitals in England and patients with dangerous, violent or criminal propensities. *Medicine, Science and the Law,* 1970, *10*(2), 93–103. (a)

Greenland, C. The three special hospitals in England and patients with dangerous, violent or criminal propensities. *Medicine, Science and the Law,* 1970, *10* (3), 180–8. (b)

Greenland, C. *Mental illness and civil liberty: A study of mental health review tribunals in England and Wales.* London: Bell, 1970. (c)

Greenland, C. *Violent offences against persons study.* Unpublished report for the Department of the Solicitor General, Ottawa 1972.

Greenland, C. Psychiatry and the dangerous sexual offender. *Canadian Psychiatric Association Journal,* 1977, *22,* 155–9.

Greenland, C. Psychiatry and the prediction of dangerousness. *Journal of Psychiatric Treatment and Evaluation,* 1980, *2,* 97–103. (a)

Greenland, C. Lethal family situations: An international comparison of deaths from child abuse. In E. J. Anthony & C. Chiland (Eds.), *The child and his family: Preventive psychiatry in an age of transition.* New York: Wiley-Interscience, 1980. (b)

Greenland, C. An experiment that failed. *Canadian Journal of Criminology,* 1984, *26*(8) 1–12.

Greenland, C., & Rosenblatt, E. *Murder followed by suicide in Ontario, 1966–1970.* Unpublished manuscript, McMaster University, 1975.

Kittrie, N. N. *The right to be different: Deviance and enforced therapy.* Baltimore: Johns Hopkins Press, 1971.

Mark, V. M., & Ervin, F. R. *Violence and the brain.* New York: Harper & Row, 1970.

McGrath, P. G. The psychiatrist's view. In J. R. Hamilton & H. Freeman (Eds.), *Dangerousness: Psychiatric assessment and management.* London: Royal College of Psychiatrists, 1982.

McKnight, C. K., Mohr, J. W., Quinsey, R. E., & Erochko, J. Matricide and mental illness. *Canadian Psychiatric Association Journal,* 1966, *11,* 99–106.

Megargee, E. I. Methodological problems in the prediction of violence. In J. R. Hays, T. K. Roberts, & K. S. Solway (Eds.), *Violence and the violent individual.* New York: Spectrum, 1981.

Mohr, J. W., Turner, R. E., & Jerry, H. B. *Pedophilia and exhibitionism.* Toronto: University of Toronto Press, 1964.

Monahan, J. *Predicting violent behavior: An assessment of clinical techniques.* Beverly Hills: Sage, 1981.

Price, R. R., & Gold, A. D. Legal controls for the dangerous offender. In *Studies of imprisonment.* Ottawa: Law Reform Commission of Canada, 1976.

Quinsey, V. L. Assessments of the dangerousness of mental patients held in maximum security. *International Journal of Law and Psychiatry,* 1979, *2,* 389–406.

Scott, P. D. Fatal battered baby cases. *Medicine, Science and Law,* 1973, *13,* 197–206.

Steadman, H. J. Special problems in the prediction of violence among the mentally ill. In J. R. Hays, T. K. Roberts, & K. S. Solway (Eds.), *Violence and the violent individual.* New York: Spectrum, 1981.

Szasz, T. S. *Law, liberty and psychiatry: An inquiry into the social uses of mental health practices.* New York: Collier, 1958.

Walker, N. Richard of Cheddestan's case. *Crime and insanity in England.* Vol. 1: *The historical perspective.* Edinburgh: University of Edinburgh Press, 1968.

Walzer, M. Timerman and his enemies. *New York Review of Books,* 1981, September 24, pp. 16–18.

Williams, D. Neural factors related to habitual aggression. *Brain,* 1969, *92*(3), 503–20.

3 Dangerous Doctor Fischer: a case history in clinical assessment?

Christopher D. Webster and Mark H. Ben-Aron

> Remember particularly that you cannot be a judge of any one. For no one can judge a criminal, until he recognises that he is just such a criminal as the man standing before him, and that he perhaps is more than all men to blame for that crime. When he understands that, he will be able to be a judge.
>
> Words of the Elder, Father Zossima
> Dostoyevsky, *The Brothers Karamazov*

Many readers of this book on the prediction of dangerousness and its implications for public policy will be expecting an exclusive emphasis on key theoretical and practical issues. Understandably, they will wonder, therefore, what the present topic might contribute to the subject at hand. Indeed, what does *Doctor Fischer of Geneva or the Bomb Party* (Greene, 1981) have to do with dangerousness? Is its author Graham Greene not only a famous novelist, but also an expert in forensic clinical assessment and the prediction of dangerousness? Do I have to read the book in order to make sense of this chapter? Because this essay does not seem to be directly related to the other chapters, should I skip it altogether? These are perfectly fair questions. In answering them, we can allay the reader's fears and at the same time introduce the rest of the chapter.

We make *Doctor Fischer of Geneva or the Bomb Party* the basis for our discussion because it allows us to present an especially interesting type of clinical case. True, the case is made up, but it is created by a writer who has something important to say to us both in a particular and in a general sense. From the general viewpoint, it must be acknowledged that Mr. Greene is a literary craftsman of the first rank. He has been affected by what he has seen in the course of a long career spent in many parts of the world. These experiences, transformed, have had their effects on a wide range of readers and an even wider range of moviegoers. He has given us such memorable characters as Henry Scoby in *The Heart of the Matter*, Mr. Wormold in *Our Man in Havana*, and Pinky in *Brighton Rock*. These people never seem like cardboard figures and never exist in isolation. They possess an abundance of human frailties, and they are cast in

41

intricate social webs. These social connections amplify the weaknesses and bring out the character. In the end the reader is often left with an altogether unexpected mixture of feelings, good and bad, for some of the most extraordinarily unsavory characters. The main actors do dreadful things, but we are induced to see them in a compassionate light.

Courts use the psychiatric remand for a variety of reasons (see Webster, Menzies, & Jackson, 1982, pp. 1–21). Beyond the strict interests of justice, they may wish to have forensic clinicians help to determine whether a compassionate view of a case is merited. Although rarely stated in such terms, it is often an important reason for an examination. As well as information about brain function and other, more conventionally scientific matters, courts expect to find out something about how patients live, how they have come to view the world, and how others now perceive them. Despite our present admitted limitations in scientific and medical knowledge, it is usually often easier to deal with these seemingly "technical" matters than with the more existential issues. Have a young mental health trainee sit in a forensic psychiatric assessment for the first time, and he or she is apt to emerge saying, "I felt so sorry for the person." Ask one of the experienced examining clinicians about the same patient and a less sympathetic answer might be forthcoming. This is not to say that the clinician is "wrong" in his view of the case; yet there exists the possibility that, with constant exposure to very difficult human problems, clinicians can and do become jaded. It is in this general sense that Mr. Greene's case becomes helpful to clinical workers. He reminds us of the subtleties involved in our complex dealings with one another and forces us to draw on a full range of emotions when we deal with our cases.

So far so good, but most of our readers will still think that we should move on as quickly as possible to the reason for including here an account of the *Bomb Party*. One or two might, as we suggested earlier, hope to learn that Mr. Greene has indeed recently taken a specialized course in clinical criminology of the kind advocated by Park Dietz in his chapter of this book. He does, however, make no such pretense, and to our certain knowledge he has not become a consultant to the Maudsley Hospital on the prediction of dangerous behavior. Yet his keen observations on human experience make him a much better guide of the affairs of the heart than most standard works of reference in psychiatry and psychology. His examples come from the real world, which, in the end, is the one we must live in. He inspires a profound appreciation of the human condition. We see ourselves in his characters. It is in exactly this sense that his works, of which the *Bomb Party* happens to be a particularly good instance, are of immense value to all those called on to undertake clinical assessments. The *Bomb Party* is a case example that clearly relies on the stuff of forensic evaluations. It analyzes intense emotions, threatened violence, psychological damage, physical injury, and death.

Mr. Greene deals with his characters and themes at many levels and in a variety of circumstances. All this is not easy to see or understand at a glance. The responses of the characters seem at times to be fairly predictable, but as we explore and understand them more deeply they are less so.

It will not be necessary for the reader to delve into Mr. Greene's book to understand the points we are trying to make. We do, of course, recommend that the book be read, if for no other reason than that, even today, it is hard to get within 150 pages one mutilation, one grizzly accidental skiing death, one suicide, one "psychological killing," and a couple of bungled suicides. The most case-hardened forensic clinician will see that this is a great value for the money. The above notwithstanding, we shall next provide a précis of the novel. Like all summaries, this cannot be expected to do justice to the original, but it should provide the reader with sufficient detail to make our chapter comprehensible. In what follows we have placed certain of our own comments and digressions in brackets.

Outline of the plot

The narrator in Mr. Greene's *Doctor Fischer of Geneva or the Bomb Party* is a widowed man in his fifties. Jones is marked by the absence of his left hand, which he lost during an explosion in the blitz of London during World War II. The son of a diplomat, he is versed in several languages and works in a chocolate factory outside Geneva. There he writes letters all day in various languages about these chocolates. He is an unassuming man who expects little from his life and counts himself fortunate that he loved his wife, whom he lost years ago through death in childbirth. But he chances to meet an attractive 20-year-old, Anna-Luise, in a cafe. They strike up a relationship, fall in love, and are soon married. The marriage is idyllic.

Anna-Luise, the young wife, has an enormously rich father, who goes by the title Doctor Fischer. What kind of doctor he is no one knows. Although he does not like it pointed out, it is common knowledge that he made his money from the invention of a toothpaste (Dentophil Bouquet). He lives by a lake in a huge, luxurious house. Like the narrator, he is widowed, Anna-Luise's mother having died some years earlier. From the outset, then, Greene is at work skillfully painting two evocative pictures in parallel. There is the doctor, rich and mysterious. Jones, in contrast, is humble but straightforward. The doctor has his title and his power over others. Jones cannot even manage to get called "mister" and considers himself lucky not to be taken for Smith. He has no authority over anyone. The doctor is a shadowy and sinister character who, well before the reader ever meets him, is surrounded by an atmosphere of evil and menace. The reader is primed to entertain all manner of horrible expectations about this "dangerous

Doctor Fisher" before the man has even uttered his first word. [In this we have an implication for the way in which bias can be introduced into clinical assessments; see, for example, Pfohl, 1978.]

Anna-Luise ascribes her mother's death directly to her father because Doctor Fischer had taken exception to an innocent relationship the mother had established with a Mr. Steiner over a shared love of music. Doctor Fischer, with his influence and wealth, ruined Mr. Steiner. Anna-Luise tells Jones that Steiner "simply disappeared." She goes on: "And my mother disappeared too after a few years. I think she was like an African who can just will herself to die" (p. 41).

The book's action centers on Doctor Fischer's personality and conduct. He has assembled around him a small group of very wealthy people who provide for him a means of "experimentation." Anna-Luise and Jones contemptuously dub these sycophants "toads." Fischer intellectualizes in an emotionally detached fashion that his cat-and-mouse games are merely exercises in studying greed, especially among the very rich. Periodically he throws parties during which he aims to humiliate his "guests," the toads, by finding out how far they will lower themselves in order to avoid losing his gifts to them. These presents, very expensive ones, come to the guests at the end of an evening of being belittled and ridiculed, but only if each obeys the doctor's dictates. As Oscar Wilde (1981) put it in "The Ballad of Reading Gaol," "Some strangle with the hands of Lust, some with the hands of Gold" (p. 668). Anna-Luise has done an assessment and dismisses her father's intellectualizations. She proffers the view that her father's abominable sadistic behavior arose because, in striking up a relationship with her mother, the inconsequential clerk Mr. Steiner "really pricked him to the heart, and he never recovered from the prick. Perhaps it was then that he learned how to *hate* and to *despise* people" (p. 41, emphasis added). [The forensic practitioner will immediately recognize the all too common themes of affection – rejection, aggression, and narcissistic assault, the mainstays of domestic violence.]

Anna-Luise greatly fears her father. When Jones suggests that he meet him before the marriage, she urges against it, saying that her father would be utterly indifferent. "If you really want to go," she says, "go, but be careful. Please be careful." Jones asks her, "Is he so dangerous?" She replies, "He's hell" (p. 18), and later she entreats him, "Please be careful and be more than ever careful if he smiles" (p. 24). Eventually, Jones is extended an invitation and, despite his wife's advice to the contrary, goes to a party where Doctor Fischer's select circle of "friends," or toads, is assembled. The party is, as expected, monstrous. In the role of cat, Doctor Fischer plays with his guests, the mice. The reader keeps expecting one of the mice to rise up against their tormentor. But this expectation, based on inadequate knowledge and understanding, is never met; the mice remain obsequious. It is this party that supplies the tension for much of the book and paves the way for the "final party." At the first party, Jones, as Doctor Fischer invariably and unceremoniously calls him, does not allow himself to be humiliated and in consequence gets no reward. The doctor says to his son-in-law, "You have a poor man's pride I see. . . . I want to discover, Jones, if the greed of our rich friends has any limit" (p. 76). Doctor Fischer's account is simplistic and almost hollow; his facade of superintelligence and power begins to tarnish. Behind his explanations we begin to glimpse a pathetic and lonely man driven by a base and false emotion. He inflicts injury on victims who are able to endure his insults only because they, too, have become slaves of their unworthy instincts. [In the unfolding analysis of his characters, Mr. Greene gives us a study of a particular kind of relationship that sometimes comes to exist between offender and victim. We refer here to the condition in which each partner is unremittingly bound to the other. The clinician will immediately see further parallels between what Mr. Greene is talking about and crimes of passion, including certain kinds of domestic violence (see D. G. Dutton, chapter 7, where we are reminded that, if we are to understand behavior of this kind we must see that it stems from emotions inculcated in the course of critical life experiences and acted out in specific contexts).]

Doctor Fischer's psychopathology continues to be carefully uncovered through his somewhat grandiose self-explanations. He tells Jones that his own greed is not for "trinkets" but likens it to God's greed, which he then with narcissistic assuredness explains. Contrary to the thought of believers and sentimentalists, God is not, according to the doctor, greedy for love. "I prefer to think that, judging from the world He is supposed to have made, He can only be greedy for our humiliation, and *that* greed how could He ever exhaust? It's bottomless" (p. 62). It is this kind of statement that causes Jones to remark to Anna-Luise, upon his return from the party, "It was revolting" and to offer to her that all-encompassing and wonderfully simple explanation: "Your father must be mad." But this is not her view. She knows better and retorts, "It would be a lot less revolting if he were" (p. 63).

In the course of the narrative, Jones and Anna-Luise chance to meet Mr. Steiner where he works in a record store. He is overcome by the sight of Anna-Luise, who closely resembles her mother. The psychological shock precipitates a heart attack. Jones later visits him in hospital, where Mr. Steiner blames himself for his entanglement with Anna-Luise's mother. He says, "It was my fault – and Mozart's . . . and her loneliness. She wasn't responsible for her loneliness." And he reveals "a touch of anger" when, referring to the doctor, he says "Perhaps he knows now what loneliness is like" (p. 73). This, as we shall see, is a key line. He muses about the dead woman: "It's strange, isn't it, she didn't love me and yet she had the will to die. I loved her and yet I didn't have enough will to die" (p. 74).

The reader is provoked by this description to wonder what the seemingly mild Mr. Steiner will do with his actually intense feelings. [Presumably, it is precisely that "touch of anger" that clinicians are expected to notice, to interpret, and if necessary to act on. In the case of Mr. Steiner, would the clinician risk a prediction about his intentions? Is he suicidal? Is he overwhelmed by feelings of hurt, sadness, and impotency? Is he homicidal, so frustrated and angry that he is on the brink of meting out revenge on the doctor? Will it be civil commitment for Mr. Steiner and/or a call to the police? Should Jones alert Doctor Fischer? In line with Bernard Dickens's chapter near the end of this book, is there a duty to warn another person of possible peril?]

Anna-Luise is killed in a skiing accident. Jones buries her. He alone is at her funeral. Although he wants sincerely to die, he cannot master the mechanics of it. A little later an opportunity presents itself. He is invited to the doctor's "final party" and he goes. The doctor has set up an elaborate outdoor dinner in the snow, including a "bran tub" containing crackers. These crackers have within them checks for huge sums of money. One cracker, however, contains a bomb. The purpose of the "experiment" is straightforward: The doctor wants to know if his toads, people who have ample money, will be ready to risk their lives for more. Again Greene's characters show us the rich mosaic of human nature that makes the clinician's job of assessment at once absorbing and difficult. The toads show their individuality and once again are predictable and unpredictable in their behavior, which is variously courageous, cowardly, selfish, and generous. But Jones, who has no further wish to live, is eager to accept the bomb-laden cracker and, eschewing the money, seeks it eagerly. When, however, he finally rips open the last cracker, which should contain the bomb, "the silly insignificant crack and the silence which followed told me how utterly I had been fooled. Doctor Fischer had stolen my death" (p. 135) – and, it might be added, finally uncovered the true shallowness and pain of his own false and meaningless existence, his lack of strength and conviction.

Away now from the party, Jones meets Mr. Steiner at the lakeside. Steiner is raging at the world. He realizes that "I had too much accepted things" (p. 137) and that, referring to the doctor, "he made innocence dirty. Now I want to get near enough to him to spit in God Almighty's face" (p. 137). He thinks that Fischer "made me what I am now" (p. 137). But Mr. Steiner does not have to seek his quarry, for the doctor himself intrudes on the two as they stand by the lake. Steiner wants to spit on Doctor Fischer. Jones wants to be dead. And the doctor, for the first time in the book, is shown in his true condition, a lonely old man at a loss for words who is despised by others and who despises himself.

[This again, it seems to us, is the stuff of which forensic psychiatric assessments are made. Who is likely to do what to whom and when? Whom should be told, and what action should be taken?]

When Jones says to the doctor, "You had your fun tonight anyway," Fischer replies, "Yes. It was better than nothing. Nothing is a bit frightening, Jones" (p. 140). The ominous Doctor Fischer is now transformed for the reader into a human character. The doctor, referring to the fact that he has for years despised himself, says, "It was a disease I caught when you came into my life, Steiner." After the doctor leaves, Steiner says to Jones, "Poor man." Jones replies "You are very charitable, Mr. Steiner. I've never hated a man more." Steiner comes back with, "You hate him and I suppose I hate him too. But hate – it isn't important. Hate isn't contagious. It doesn't spread. One can hate one man and leave it there. But when you begin to despise like Doctor Fischer, you end by despising all the world" (p. 141). The two man then hear a shot as Doctor Fischer kills himself.

Mr. Steiner's lines about the difference between hating and despising have a bearing on the present topic that is too obvious to warrant extended discussion. Both Jones and Mr. Steiner have the capacity to love but, though wishing death, cannot destroy themselves. In concluding his narrative, Jones notes "unlike Doctor Fischer, I never found the courage necessary to kill myself; that night [of the bomb party] I hadn't needed courage, for I had a sufficiency of despair" (p. 142). He goes on, "Courage is sapped by day-to-day mind-dulling routine, and despair deepens so much every day one lives, that death seems in the end to lose its point" (p. 142).

The *Bomb Party* and clinical assessment

As they do their forensic psychiatric assessments, clinicians should surely find in their patients and in themselves something of the same emotional fuels that propel Mr. Greene's characters. A degree of identification with the patient is called for if these driving forces are to be analyzed and understood. The job is to create an impression of the person from whatever written material lies at hand and whatever information the person chooses to give. Clinicians are limited by their intelligence, by their idiosyncratic biases, and at times even by their professional jargon. Thoughtful researchers like Megargee (1976) offer us the beginning of a new vocabulary adequate for the task of predicting dangerous behavior. The need for this is addressed by Dr. Martin in chapter 5. Such terms as "instigation to aggression," "angry aggression," and "instrumental aggression" in Megargee's definitional scheme, although obviously lacking the subtle nuances found in the work of a writer like Mr. Greene, offer some prospect. As an example, "angry aggression," a term advanced by Buss (1961), can be defined as being "motivated by a conscious or unconscious desire to harm the victim and is reinforced by the victim's pain," whereas "instrumental aggression" is "a means to some other end and is reinforced by the satisfaction of some other drive" (p. 7). Shooting someone one hates is an example of angry aggression; shooting someone in self-defense or under contract is an example of instrumental aggression. This "explanation" poses another question. What was Doctor Fischer's conscious or unconscious desire? As tools to unravel the matter farther, let us refer to Megargee's terms "hostility" and "anger." Megargee tells us, "Hostility is a relatively enduring characteristic or trait, whereas anger or rage are transitory emotional states which are highly individualized and situation-specific" (p. 7). We can now say that Dr. Fischer's behavior was motivated by angry aggression and that he is hostile. But again, we wonder whether this word "hostility," grossly overused in clinical practice, offers any real enlightenment. Megargee sees this point clearly. He notes that the "vast majority of psycho-metric devices available simply attempt to measure aggressive motivation (or worse yet, 'aggressiveness') as though they were enduring traits" (p. 7). He goes on to say, however, that the case history and interviews with family and friends are apt to yield the most useful information with which to assess the potential for future dangerous behavior. Mr. Greene has given us a case history with family and friends bound by emotions and circumstances not especially different from those typically seen in everyday lives. Love, hate, pain, pleasure, despair, likes, dislikes, fears, wants, desires are all present and active.

He shows what might be accomplished if we could but make the effort to use words to uncover successively the "layers" each person uses for protection from the world be he or she prisoner, patient, or clinician. It takes training and persistence to learn how to use a microscope. At first, the untutored eye sees mere blobs of matter. Only gradually does the student learn to separate the mass into specific entities, to name the structures, and to see the connections between them. Similarly, it requires experience and effort to conduct clinical interviews with care and imagination. The interview is as important as the microscope and is of just as much interest from a scientific point of view.

This much said, it is nonetheless difficult for any of us to identify fully our own emotional states. Genius may be required to infer the emotional condition of another. Jones tells Doctor Fischer that he despises him. The doctor retorts, "Again you are using the wrong term. Semantics are important, Jones. I tell you, you hate, you don't despise. To despise comes out of a great disappointment. . . . When one despises, Jones, it's like a deep and incurable wound, the beginning of death. And one must revenge one's wound while there's still time. When the one who inflicted it is dead, one has to strike back at others" (p. 105). This leads Jones to another attempt to "label" the doctor. He says, "Perhaps you are right, Fischer. Perhaps I shouldn't even hate you. I think you are mad"

(p. 106). But just as Anna-Luise had earlier discerned, the madness theory is altogether too crude to be applied to the doctor. " 'Oh no, no, not mad,' he said with that small unbearable smile of ineffable superiority'' (p. 106) and goes on in the next breath to remind us that it is not everyone who can call another mad: "It's amusing to watch how they react. None of them [the toads] would dare to call me mad as you have done. They might lose an invitation to my next party'' (p. 106).

If Doctor Fischer is not mad, then what is it that prompts his efforts to humiliate and destroy others? What "diagnosis" covers him best? Doctor Fischer is by no means unintelligent. He knows his condition and that of those around him. "Money makes a difference certainly. Some people will even die for money, Jones. They don't die for love except in novels'' (p. 107). This statement causes Jones himself to reflect: "I thought I had tried to do just that, and was it for love I had tried or was it from the fear of an irremediable loneliness?'' (p. 107). Jones is making the assessment. Fischer is the assessee. But Jones cannot hope to reach a final and "accurate" opinion of the doctor until Fischer's predicament comes to have some actual bearing on him. Jones cannot "see" or even begin to appreciate the doctor until he works out a suitable emotional reaction toward him. Somehow Jones has got to find empathy for the doctor. He must find a way of analyzing and describing the doctor's emotions. In some measure he must be able to place himself in the framework of the doctor's existence. By the end of the book the author has achieved his purpose in explaining for us, through Jones, the roots of the doctor's intolerable but not actually incomprehensible conduct.

Although we do not wish to denigrate our own hard efforts to define the kinds of emotional states that underlie some aspects of dangerous behavior or to find ways of yielding the necessary intercoder agreements so admirably called for in the next two chapters, it is nonetheless obvious that this essentially reductionist kind of approach has, if we are to follow Mr. Greene, considerable practical limitations. Small wonder, perhaps, that we "account for but a fraction of the total variance.'' Vernon Quinsey (1975) once put it well in reminding us that dangerousness is not only a matter of "external criteria" (such as type of offense), but as well "a social judgment and related to the characteristics of the observers" (p. 66). Unless we are careful, the patient is "other," "out there," "removed,'' and it is unrealistic to expect that we as experts can, through the use of specialized instruments (such as the *Diagnostic and Statistical Manual of Mental Disorders*, 1980), pin down the condition. Now we do not wish here to enter into a polemic against psychiatric classification. This is a complex matter, one dealt with fully by Dr. Martin in chapter 5. Our point, based on the *Bomb Party*, is that, if indeed we ever do take seriously Dr. Dietz's suggestion to train people to assess potential for dangerousness, the assessor's reaction to threatening conditions must be taken into account. We can clarify this point a little by

returning one last time to the *Bomb Party*. During the time that Jones is waiting
for Anna-Luise to ski back down the mountain, he "buys" a window table from
a disagreeable waiter. When, eventually, he returns to the hotel after Anna-Luise
is brought down on a stretcher in a coma, the waiter is "more surly than ever."
The waiter says, "You reserved this table for lunch. I have had to turn away
customers." Jones retorts, "There's one customer you'll never see again." He
throws a fifty-centime piece on the table, which falls on the floor. "Then I waited
by the door to see if he would pick it up. He did and I felt ashamed. But if it had
been in my power *I would have revenged myself for what had happened on all
the world* – like Doctor Fischer, I thought, just like Doctor Fischer" (p. 91,
emphasis added). At that precise moment Jones could understand Doctor Fischer
and could, perhaps, begin to predict his behavior. Whereas Jones has been the
assessor throughout and the doctor the person evaluated, we see the positions
suddenly reversed and, in the shift, a clarification. Clinicians must surely use
themselves as the microscope. They must look at human frailties and can understand the extent of others' shortcomings only if they know their own. This point
has been well put in the dangerousness literature by Hershel Prins (1981): "In
order to operate effectively and humanely in work with dangerous and potentially
dangerous offenders, it is therefore necessary to have tried to come to terms with
one's own potential for violent or dangerous behaviour" (p. 130).

The *Bomb Party* is about hating, detesting, despising, fearing, humiliating,
and loving. It deals with pride, contempt, cruelty, and courage. Although ad-
mirable definitions of these words can be found in the *Shorter Oxford,* they are
in fact, despite their everyday currency, difficult to use when it comes to con-
veying as precisely as possible one's own emotional state, let alone that of another person. In our greatly needed attempts to create technical vocabularies[1] for
the assessment of dangerousness, it seems to us that the English language, properly used as it is in the hands of Graham Greene, can inspire us to greater attempts at clarity and precision in our assessing and our predicting.

Note

1 Monahan (1981) adopts the Megargee outlook as far as personality variables are concerned and
   directs us to Novaco (1975) for a discussion about the assessment of anger, but he also notes:
   "Affective reactions inhibiting violence (or, to put it more positively, predisposing toward peace-
   fulness) include what have been called the 'moral emotions' of empathy for the source of a frustration and guilt about injuring another, as well as anxiety reactions about engaging in violence or
   about the victim's possible retaliation" (p. 155). It seems to us that novelists like Greene know a
   good deal about the "moral emotions."

References

Buss, A. H. *Psychology of aggression*. New York: Wiley, 1961.
Diagnostic and Statistical Manual of Mental Disorders (3rd ed.). Washington, D.C.: American
    Psychiatric Association.

Greene, G. *Doctor Fischer of Geneva or the bomb party*. Harmondsworth, Middlesex: Penguin, 1981.

Megargee, E. I. The Prediction of dangerous behavior. *Criminal Justice and Behavior,* 1976, *3,* 3–21.

Monahan, J. *Predicting violent behavior: An assessment of clinical techniques*. Beverly Hills: Sage, 1981.

Novaco, R. *Anger control: The development and evaluation of an experimental treatment*. Lexington, Mass: Lexington Books, 1975.

Pfohl, S. *Predicting dangerousness: The social construction of psychiatric reality*. Lexington, Mass.: Heath, 1978.

Prins, H. A. Dangerous people or dangerous situations? Some implications for assessment and management. *Medicine Science and Law,* 1981, *21,* 125–33.

Quinsey, V. L. Psychiatric staff conferences on dangerous mentally disordered offenders. *Canadian Journal of Behavioural Science,* 1975, *7,* 60–9.

Webster, C. D., Menzies, R. J., & Jackson, M. A. *Clinical assessment before trial: Legal issues and mental disorder*. Toronto: Butterworths, 1982.

Wilde, O. The ballad of Reading Gaol. In R. Addington & S. Weintraub (Eds.), *The portable Oscar Wilde* (rev. ed.). Harmondsworth, Middlesex: Penguin, 1981.

4 The predictive value of the clinical assessment for the diagnosis, prognosis, and treatment response of patients

R. Brian Haynes

Depending on the nature of the disorder and the diagnostic tools available, the diagnosis and/or management plan for most individuals with physical or mental disorders can or must be made on the basis of the clinical assessment. Sandler (1979) has shown, for example, that an accurate diagnosis can be established for 56% of patients at a general medical clinic on the basis of the physician's historical inquiry alone, and an additional 17% can be diagnosed when the results of the physical examination are added to those of the inquiry. For mental diseases, of course, virtually all diagnosis and management must depend on the clinical assessment.

However, in an era of many highly precise, quantitative diagnostic tests we have become suspicious of the reliability of clinical assessment and are in some danger of undermining its validity through a misunderstanding of its role and through a neglect of the principles and practice required to optimize reliability and validity.

This chapter provides some examples of the potency and impotency of various clinical observations, describes some basic principles for the evaluation and proper interpretation of clinical information, and proposes some tasks that each clinical discipline might take on to improve its collection and use of clinical information. The term "use" is applied somewhat narrowly here to include only the predictive value of clinical observations for the diagnosis, prognosis, and therapeutic responsiveness of the patient. There are, no doubt, other uses of clinical assessments that merit consideration but do not receive it here.

The predictive value of the clinical assessment

The first step in clinical encounters is to collect data by questioning patients (if that is possible) and by examining them physically. Generally, the initial assess-

53

ment is somewhat preliminary and is used to predict a diagnosis that will be established more definitively by various tests or in the course of time. Less frequently, the clinical work-up can be used to predict the response of a patient to a given treatment or to anticipate the patient's general course. Examples of these uses are hardly necessary, but the following will illustrate the strength of some very simple clinical observations.

The likelihood that a person has coronary artery disease can be determined with a high degree of accuracy on the basis of his or her age, sex, and symptoms alone. A 60-year-old male patient with "typical angina" (exertional retrosternal chest pain relieved within 5 to 15 min by rest) has a 94.3% likelihood of being found to have significant coronary atherosclerosis (with at least 75% occlusion of at least one coronary artery) on angiography, whereas a 30-year-old woman with nonanginal chest pain has only a 0.8% chance of a similar finding (Diamond & Forrester, 1979). Angiography in the man's case would be indicated only if surgical intervention were being contemplated, a diagnosis having been established about as certainly from the clinical circumstances as it would be reasonable to desire, particularly considering the risk of angiography.

In the woman's situation, it would be difficult to justify angiography because its risk of inducing complications exceeds the likelihood that she has coronary artery disease. If she is worried about a heart attack, she should be exuberantly reassured and sent home. Although we have a plethora of noninvasive tests that could be applied in such situations, they are quite unnecessary for diagnostic purposes, given the extreme "pretest likelihood" of disease, and might even be misleading (Department of Clinical Epidemiology and Biostatistics, 1981a).

As for prognosis, Boyd and Feinstein (1978) have shown that the survival of patients with Hodgkin's disease can be predicted more accurately from the patient's symptoms at the time of diagnosis than from the traditional Ann Arbor Staging System, which requires surgical exploration with biopsy of various lymphatic and extralymphatic tissues.

The likelihood of responsiveness to therapy can also be predicted from simple clinical observations. For example, among patients with transient ischemic attacks or partial strokes, the risk of recurrence can be reduced by 50% in men by regular aspirin ingestion, but women do not respond to this treatment at all (Canadian Stroke Study Cooperative Group, 1978).

The strength of the clinical observations described here is undeniable, although I would conjecture that few clinicians are aware of the degree of accuracy of such observations in prediction and fewer still apply them to advantage. At the same time, many clinical observations that lack value are slavishly recorded. For example, the jugular venous pressure cannot be reliably assessed on clinical examination of patients with respiratory disorders, even after considerable practice (Godfrey, Edwards, & Campbell, 1969). Indeed, the reliability and predictive value of many clinical assessments are unknown, a sad state of affairs when one considers the potential value of some clinical findings, the potential inadequacy of others, and the extraordinary amount of time that clinicians spend collecting these data. Who can doubt that patients would be better served and practitioners would make better use of their time if the predictive value of clinical observations were known and if those with low or no value were deleted to permit more careful attention to those that had a measurable relationship to important patient outcomes? The remainder of this chapter explores the scientific concepts that apply to the determination of the value of clinical observations. This approach is generated by the premise that most clinicians do not understand these concepts clearly and the belief that knowledge of the concepts can enhance clinical competency and, thus, patient care.

Determining the reliability and accuracy of clinical assessment

Clinical observations are subject to inaccuracy, unreliability, and bias. These three terms have rather specific meanings in the argot of measurement science and merit elaboration. Inaccuracy occurs when the clinical assessment fails to give the true clinical value, as determined by some external "gold standard." For example, when house officers assess fetal heart rates by stethoscope, they tend to report the rate as higher than it actually is by fetal heart monitor when the true rate is lower than normal, and they report it as lower than it actually is when the fetal heart rate is high (Day, Maddern, & Wood, 1968). As a second example, a patient's true level of compliance with a medication regime can be determined by serum drug levels and other means, but when physicians are asked to rate their patients as compliant or noncompliant, they are no more accurate than would be a monkey flipping a coin (Gilbert et al., 1980).

Unreliability is quite a different matter. A clinical measurement method is unreliable when repeated applications of it to the same attribute by the same clinician or by different clinicians fail to give the same results. Unreliability in the same clinician is referred to as intraobserver variation and that in different clinicians, interobserver variation. Synonyms for unreliability include unreproducibility, imprecision, and inconsistency. Examples of unreliability are legion in clinical practice. After considerable experience and a period of special training in which terminology and definitions were standardized, Beck et al. (1962) found that agreement among psychiatrists on diagnoses was only 43% better than would be expected on the basis of chance alone. This was considerably higher than the degree of reliability found in the previous studies, in less pristine circumstances, that these investigators reviewed. Intraobserver variation is less than interobserver variation but is still often considerable. For example, intraobserver agreement in examining optic fundi was found to be 68% over chance, whereas inter-observer agreement between two ophthalmologists examining the same fundi was 55% over chance (Aoki et al., 1977).

Although virtually all clinical assessments are unreliable to a degree, most that have been studied to date are demonstrably more reliable than would be expected if the assessments were entirely haphazard, and it has been shown that unreliability can be reduced by a variety of tactics such as defining criteria and comparing notes with one's colleagues. For example, Godfrey et al. (1969) demonstrated that interobserver agreement for physical signs could be improved from 59 to 70% by a 1-month period of conferring among colleagues on specific cases.

The relationship between unreliability and inaccuracy is important but somewhat complex. First, an assessment that is unreliable cannot be accurate because the relationship between a given assessment and the true value cannot be specified. A reliable assessment, however, is not necessarily accurate. A common analogy here is that of the good marksman whose gunsight is off; his shots will be grouped closely together (i.e., reliable) but away from the center of the target (i.e., inaccurate). This is generally a much more favorable situation than that of the poor marksman whose shots are scattered (unreliable), even though he may occasionally score a bull's-eye, because the good marksman's shots can be made accurate by a simple adjustment of the gunsight. The magnitude of this adjustment is called "bias" (defined as the systematic alteration of an assessment from the true value being measured), and it is a useful concept in many clinical assessments. For example, if patients are asked to estimate their compliance with a prescribed medication regime, those who are less than fully compliant will generally overestimate their compliance by an amount that averages about 20% (Haynes et al., 1980). Thus, if one wishes to know which of one's patients are taking less than 80% of their medication, the question should be phrased, "Do you ever miss *any* of your pills?" (Haynes et al., 1980). A second example is one given earlier concerning the tendency of house officers to "normalize" extreme values of fetal heart rates (Day et al., 1968).

In clinical medicine there are some additional important features of accuracy, reliability, and bias. First, for many clinical assessments no "gold standard" of accuracy exists. For example, there is no electronic gizmo that can be applied to a patient's pate to ascertain his or her affective state. The evaluation of the patient must be clinical (depression rating scales being simply standardized surrogates for the clinical assessment). Neither the accuracy nor the bias of these assessments can be measured. We are left, then, with reliability as the only measure of the worth of such assessments. Although this state of affairs is not very satisfactory, at least reliability is a concept worth hanging our hats on. Recalling that assessments with low reliability must have, at best, low accuracy, the imperative is to improve the reliability of these clinical measures to the extent that is humanly possible.

Second, reliable and accurate assessments are not necessarily worthwhile. For example, a machine can reliably and accurately assess the level of sodium in one's plasma. However, the plasma sodium level bears no constant relationship to the amount of sodium in the body, and clinical assessments, indisputably less accurate and reliable than the plasma sodium level determination, are required to interpret the import (or lack of it) of the sodium value. Thus, one might distinguish between what is important to measure and what one can measure well. Although we would all wish to live in a clinical world in which all important phenomena could be measured accurately, it would be folly to forego a somewhat unreliable (but not thoroughly so) clinical measurement of an important phenomenon for a highly accurate measure of an unimportant one or one that applied to only one facet of the patient's clinical state. Nevertheless, clinically, we do this regularly in many ways. For example, in treating hypertensive patients, clinicians might prescribe weight reduction, salt restriction, moderate exercise, and one or more pills to be taken daily for an eternity. To measure the effect of this treatment program we assess the patient's blood pressure, but what about the quality of the patient's life? Although we might appreciate the magnitude of the changes we are asking the patient to make (particularly if we have had to cope with such a regimen personally), we would seldom attempt to measure the effect. If we did measure the effect on the patient, using any one of a number of (somewhat) reliable quality-of-life scales, we might be able to achieve a better compromise between the patient's blood pressure and his or her joie de vivre. But few clinicians know anything about such assessments. (Indeed, they barely do a passable job of measuring blood pressure.)

It is beyond the scope of this chapter to delve into the sources of error in clinical assessment or the means of remedying them; the interested reader is referred to another source (Department of Clinical Epidemiology and Biostatistics, 1980a, 1980b). The main point is that error does exist in clinical assessment but it can often be measured, analyzed, and ameliorated.

Determining the predictive value of clinical assessments

Reliability is a measure of the intrinsic variability of a measurement, whereas accuracy is a measure of the extrinsic validity of a measurement. Predictive value, in the context in which it is described in this chapter, is a subset of accuracy and refers to the capacity of a clinical assessment to predict a clinically important event, whether this be the establishment of a diagnosis by a (more) definitive test, the response of the patient to therapy, or the prognosis of the patient. Some examples of the predictive value of clinical assessments for diagnosis, prognosis, and therapeutic response were given earlier, and now we turn to some of the concepts that are important for determining predictive value.

Table 4.1 provides a fairly simple way to depict the principles. Above the

Table 4.1. *"Blind" comparison of clinical assessment with an objective measure of outcome*

Clinical assessment	Outcome measure[a]		
	Patient has outcome	Patient does not have outcome	
Positive: Patient appears to be at risk of outcome	a	b	$a+b$
Negative	c	d	$c+d$
	$a+c$	$b+d$	$a+b+c+d$

Note: Stable properties: $a/(a+c)$ = sensitivity; $d/(b+d)$ = specificity. Prevalence-dependent properties: $a/(a+b)$ = positive predictive value; $d/(c+d)$ = negative predictive value; $(a+d)/(a+b+c+d)$ = accuracy.
[a] Outcome refers to the establishment of a definitive diagnosis or the occurrence of a therapeutic response or the determination of prognosis.
Source: Adapted from Department of Clinical Epidemiology and Biostatistics (1981a).

columns of the two-by-two table are the clinical states to be predicted, whether they be diagnosis, prognosis, or treatment response, as established in the course of time by some acceptable standard. Beside the rows of the table are the results of the clinical assessment under scrutiny. If a group of patients with a given complaint are evaluated by *both* the clinical assessment and the standard, then the cells in the table can be filled in. Ideally, all patients would fall in the upper left-hand cell or lower right-hand cell, indicating perfect agreement, but under usual circumstances the remaining two cells would be occupied as well.

The two-by-two arrangement can be analyzed in a bewildering variety of ways, but for our purposes the approach has been standardized and labels have been given to the various calculations, as noted in the table (for details, see Department of Clinical Epidemiology and Biostatistics, 1981a). The key points are these. First, sensitivity and specificity are regarded as "stable" properties in that they remain constant for a given clinical assessment and clinical state. By contrast, the positive and negative predictive values and accuracy of the clinical assessment are affected by the prevalence of the abnormal clinical state. The consequence of this is that practitioners must know three things in order to interpret the clinical findings correctly. First, they must know the sensitivity of their assessment (i.e., its capacity to detect those patients with the clinical state of interest). Second, they must know the specificity of their assessment (i.e., its

Table 4.2. *Prediction of therapeutic responsiveness in a weight reduction program*

A. Actual study

Clinical feature	Completed program		Total
	No	Yes	
Smoker	18	10	28
Nonsmoker	15	37	52
Total	33	47	80

Prevalence = 33/80 = .41
Sensitivity = 18/33 = .55
Specificity = 37/47 = .78
Positive predictive value = 18/28 = .64
Negative predictive value = 37/52 = .71

B. Effect of change in "prevalence"
    of failure to complete program

Clinical feature	Completed program		Total
	No	Yes	
Smoker	9	13	22
Nonsmoker	7	51	58
Total	16	64	80

Prevalence = 16/80 = .20
Positive predictive value = 9/22 = .41
Negative predictive value = 51/58 = .88

Source: Streja et al. (1982).

capacity to identify correctly those people who are free of the abnormal clinical state). Third, they must know the prevalence of the abnormal clinical state among people who come to them (i.e., the likelihood that a given person has the abnormal clinical state). With the knowledge of all three factors, sensitivity, specificity, and prevalence, the clinicians will be able to estimate the predictive value of their findings.

Examples of predictive value are displayed in Tables 4.2 and 4.3. The "therapeutic responsiveness" of candidates for a weight reduction program was determined by Streja, Boyko, and Rabkin (1982) (Table 4.2A). In their program, the likelihood of failure of completion for those who entered was (33/80 =) 41% (i.e., prevalence). However, simply taking into account the smoking history of a patient made it possible to make a much more individualized estimate of the likelihood of failure: Smokers had a (18/28 =) 64% chance of failure (positive

Table 4.3. *Predictive value of exertional chest pain*
for angina pectoris

A. Actual study[a]

| | Final diagnosis | | |
| | Angina | Not angina | |
Clinical assessment	pectoris	pectoris	Total
Pain increased by exertion	171	292	463
Pain not increased by exertion	38	499	537
Total	209	791	1000

Prevalence = .21
Sensitivity = .82
Specificity = .63
Positive predictive value = .37
Negative predictive value = .93

B. Effect of change of prevalence of angina pectoris

| | Final diagnosis | | |
| | Angina | Not angina | |
Clinical assessment	pectoris	pectoris	Total
Pain increased by exertion	410	185	595
Pain not increased by exertion	90	315	405
Total	500	500	1000

Prevalence = .50
Positive predictive value = .69
Negative predictive value = .78

[a] Adapted from Pipberger et al. (1968).

predictive value), whereas nonsmokers had only a (15/52 =) 29% risk of failure.
If modifications were made to the program that affected smokers and nonsmokers
equally (say, through introducing a contingency charge), these predictive values
would change in calculable fashion. For example, if the dropout rate decreased
to 20%, the likelihood that a smoker would drop out would decrease to 41%
(Table 4.2B).

In the second example (Table 4.3A), Pipberger, Klingeman, and Cosma (1968)
followed patients admitted to hospital with chest pain for whom the final diagnosis could be firmly established. All patients were questioned in a standardized
fashion concerning whether the pain was increased by exertion. Among all pa-

Table 4.4. *Methodological guides in performing studies of the predictive value of clinical assessment*

Patient selection: "inception cohort"
Clinical assessment: reproducibly described; feasible in other settings
Comparisons: all patients assessed by both clinical and outcome measures
Blindness: independent, objective measure of outcome
Follow-up: all entered patients accounted for
Analysis: agreement over chance; estimate of variance

Source: Adapted from Department of Clinical Epidemiology and Biostatistics (1981a, 1981b).

tients with chest pain, 21% were ultimately found to have angina pectoris (prevalence), whereas among patients who reported that their pain was increased by exertion, the likelihood of angina was 37% (positive predictive value). In this example, although exertional chest pain is generally regarded as the sine qua non of angina pectoris and 82% of patients with angina in this study complained of it (sensitivity), the prevalence and specificity of this symptom are low enough that its presence in a patient's symptomatology by no means establishes the diagnosis. In contrast, a person who had it was (positive predictive value /[1 − negative predictive value] = 37%/7% =) 5.3 times as likely to have angina as one who did not. Table 4.3B again illustrates the profound influence of prevalence. If the proportion of patients with chest pain who are found to have angina is increased to 50% (say, by screening out of consideration people who are unlikely to have angina such as young women and people with an obvious acute cause for their chest pain such as a recent rib fracture or pneumonia), then the predictive value of having exertional chest pain increases dramatically to 69%.

This model of evaluation can be applied to any form of clinical assessment, provided that an acceptable external standard of diagnosis, prognosis, or therapeutic response is available. However, the validity and quality of such evaluations depend to an important extent on adherence to scientific principles such as described in Table 4.4. First, the sample of patients chosen should be an "inception cohort" of individuals selected, at a common point in their illness, by criteria that are reproducible by others (Department of Clinical Epidemiology, 1981a, 1981b). Second, the method of clinical assessment must be described in a reproducible fashion and must be feasible in other settings. Third, all patients included in the investigation must be assessed both clinically and by objective outcome measures (whether these be diagnostic tests or a measure of treatment response or prognosis). Fourth, outcome measures should be applied without knowledge of the clinical assessment (i.e., "blind") to avoid bias. Fifth, all patients included in the study must be accounted for. Sixth, extraneous prognostic factors should be adjusted for in the analysis. Appropriate analytic techniques should be applied that provide not simply the correlation between clinical and outcome measures, but the degree of agreement over and above that expected by chance as well as the variance of the estimate of agreement (Department of Clinical Epidemiology and Biostatistics, 1980a, 1980b). Cohen's kappa is one such statistic (Fleiss, 1973).

The scope of evaluation of the predictive value of clinical assessments can be as broad as one has measures to support. For example, an evaluation can be quite traditional and examine the agreement between clinical findings and roentgenograms or branch out and scrutinize the predictive value for quality of life or health services utilization and so on.

Strengths and limitations of the model

Potentially, a thorough evaluation of all items of clinical assessment could result in many clinical measurements being discarded as unreliable or inaccurate and in other assessments being improved or utilized in a more appropriate fashion. The need for many expensive and/or invasive diagnostic tests could be reduced, treatments could be tailored better to a patient's characteristics, and the clinician could provide the patient with an accurate estimate of his or her course. Applied to the individual clinician in training or practice, assessment of individual reliability and ability to predict outcomes from clinical findings would be a potent tool in assessing competence and performance.

Alas, we are far from realizing these goals. Despite the fact that error in clinical assessment is measurable and frequently remediable, most clinicians would be hard-pressed to provide an accurate figure of the magnitude of error in various assessments, and virtually none would be able to provide a figure of the reliability and accuracy of their own assessments. Scientists and consumers of health services would no doubt find this appalling if they were aware of it. From the clinical perspective, however, there are many mitigating considerations. To begin with, there is little in the education of clinicians that prepares them for being systematically critical about clinical skills. Second, studies of clinical assessments are generally so replete with detail that no one could possibly remember them. Third, if clinicians make mistakes but order diagnostic tests routinely, they may be put back on the right track. Fourth, if the patient fails to respond to a treatment, the clinician can always reevaluate the situation. Fifth, if patients think that their clinician is on the wrong track, they can take their problems elsewhere, and their clinician will be none the wiser. Sixth, in discussing prognosis with patients it is safer and easier to be vague or noncommittal. Seventh, it is difficult logistically for clinicians to check their own competence and performance. Eighth, clinicians lack the time to examine their clinical assessments directly or vicariously (even though they might believe that it would be the "right thing" to do and might improve their efficiency in the long run). And so on and so on.

These objections can be dismissed, for the most part, as rationalizations, but there are some serious difficulties with existing data on the value of clinical assessments. In the first place, many of the evaluations are not sound because of faulty patient selection and characterization, inadequate research design, improper application of external standards, and a host of other problems. Second, in order to make sense of clinical assessments many simplifying assumptions have to be made. The assumption about the constancy of sensitivity and specificity is one of these. Another is focusing attention on one small part of the clinical assessment when there are many parts that may be inextricably intertwined. Third, there is the immensity of the task of evaluating all clinical assessments against all clinical outcomes.

Many of these problems, however, are tractable. Some of the methodological principles necessary for their solution are understood (Department of Clinical Epidemiology and Biostatistics 1980a, 1980b, 1981a, 1981b), and work in this field has led to the formation of organizations concerned with clinical decision making using an expanding body of literature on the predictive value of clinical information. Furthermore, modern computers not only can handle the complicated tasks but, in some situations, are already becoming the companion of the stethoscope.

These developments will make life both easier and more difficult for clinicians. Good science can make clinical work easier through data reduction, the sorting out of the wheat from the chaff in clinical assessment. However, the demand for reliability in clinical assessment and the tools to assess reliability and accuracy of the individual clinician will place a higher demand for excellence on clinicians. We and our patients have more to gain than lose from this, and we must neither refuse nor procrastinate in taking up the challenge.

References

Aoki, N., Horibe, H., Ohno, Y., Hayakawa, N., Kondo, R., & Okado, H. Epidemiological evaluation in funduscopic findings in cerebrovascular diseases. 3. Observer variability and reproducibility for funduscopic findings. *Japanese Circulation Journal*, 1977, *41*, 11–17.

Beck, A. T., Ward, C. H., Mendelson, M., Mock, J. E., & Erbaugh, J. K. Reliability of psychiatric diagnosis. 2. A study of the consistency of clinical judgments and ratings. *American Journal of Psychiatry*, 1962, *119*, 351–7.

Boyd, N. R., & Feinstein, A. R. Symptoms as an index of growth rates and prognosis in Hodgkin's disease. *Clinical and Investigative Medicine*, 1978, *1*, 25–31.

Canadian Stroke Study Cooperative Group. A randomized trial of aspirin and sulfinpyrazone in threatened stroke. *New England Journal of Medicine*, 1978, *299*, 53–9.

Day, E., Maddern, L., & Wood, C. Auscultation of the foetal heart rate: An assessment of its error and significance. *British Medical Journal*, 1968, *4*, 422–4.

Department of Clinical Epidemiology and Biostatistics. Clinical disagreement. 1. How often it occurs and why. *Canadian Medical Association Journal*, 1980, *123*, 499–504. (a)

Department of Clinical Epidemiology and Biostatistics. Clinical disagreement. 2. How to avoid it and learn from one's mistakes. *Canadian Medical Association Journal*, 1980, *123*, 613–617. (b)

Department of Clinical Epidemiology and Biostatistics. How to read clinical journals. 2. To learn about a diagnostic test. *Canadian Medical Association Journal*, 1981, *124*, 703–10. (a)

Department of Clinical Epidemiology and Biostatistics. How to read clinical journals. 3. To learn about the clinical course and prognosis of disease. *Canadian Medical Association Journal*, 1981, *124*, 869–72. (b)

Diamond, G. A., & Forrester, J. S. Analysis of probability as an aid in the clinical diagnosis of coronary-artery disease. *New England Journal of Medicine*, 1979, *300*, 1350–58.

Fleiss, J. L. *Statistical methods for rates and proportions*. New York: Wiley, 1973.

Gilbert, J. R., Evans, C. E., Haynes, R. B., & Tugwell, P. Predicting compliance with a regimen of digoxin therapy in family practice. *Canadian Medical Association Journal*, 1980, *123*, 119–22.

Godfrey, S., Edwards, H., & Campbell, E. J. Repeatability of physical signs in airways obstruction. *Thorax*, 1969, *24*, 4–9.

Haynes, R. B., Taylor, D. W., Sackett, D. L., Gibson, E. S., Bernholz, C. D., & Mukherjee, J. Can simple clinical measurements detect patient compliance. *Hypertension*, 1980, *2*, 757–64.

Pipberger, H. V., Klingeman, J. D., & Cosma, J. Computer evaluation of the statistical properties of clinical information in the differential diagnosis of chest pain. *Methods of Information in Medicine*, 1968, *7*, 79–92.

Sandler, G. Cost of unnecessary tests. *British Medical Journal*, 1979, *2*, 21–4.

Streja, D. A., Boyko, E., & Rabkin, S. W. Predictors of outcome in a risk factor intervention trial using behavior modification. *Preventive Medicine*, 1982, *11*, 291–303.

5   The reliability of psychiatric diagnosis

Barry A. Martin

In chapter 4, Haynes gives us a glimpse of the medical netherworld of unreliable clinical observation and therapeutic misadventure. He provides the kind of information that might at once comfort and disturb psychiatrists. The small comfort that we are no worse than the rest of the medical specialists gives way to the uneasiness that perhaps none of us is really very good. In places, Haynes's text calls to mind thoughts about Paddy Chayefsky's screenplay for *The Hospital,* a tragicomedy of medical errors, and a memorable scene with George C. Scott reciting a litany of torts through which "the entire machinery of modern medicine has conspired to kill one lousy patient" and prudently concluding, "Let him go before we kill him."

Quite understandably, we prefer not to dwell morbidly on this aspect of medical practice lest we become too cynical. Nevertheless, the critical examination of error remains a cornerstone of continuing medical education to improve diagnostic accuracy – this notwithstanding the debate in the *New England Journal of Medicine* regarding the value of the clinical pathological conference (Lipkin, 1979; Scully, 1979). In what follows I discuss a rather fundamental area of psychiatric practice and the problems encountered therein. Although the chapter might have been more correctly titled "The Unreliability of Psychiatric Diagnosis," I would prefer not to give undue emphasis to the negative but rather to extrapolate from Haynes's encouraging comment that diagnostic reliability may be substantially improved by the development of standard defining criteria for the diagnoses we employ. It used to be said, and still is in legal circles, that three psychiatrists examining the same patient at the same time will arrive at three different diagnoses. Using standard diagnostic criteria and terminology, they are much more likely to concur. Even if their understanding or treatment of the patient and his or her disease is not any better, I would suggest that this is progress.

Before we proceed, a rhetorical question might place the issue of diagnostic reliability in perspective. What does a reliable diagnosis have to do with probability and the prediction of dangerous or antisocial behavior, the topic of this book? In the forensic psychiatry context, the diagnosis is a conclusory statement and is of limited usefulness in determining culpability or in making a prognosis with respect to the recurrence of specific behavior. It is my opinion that both the clinical and the statistical prediction of dangerous behavior should be based more on specific symptoms or discrete behaviors than on more global diagnostic categories. Notwithstanding this opinion, reliable diagnosis is dependent on reliable observation of symptoms and behavior such that the question does not obviate that which follows.

Reliability and validity

It is necessary at the outset to clarify the terms in the title of this chapter. "Reliability" simply refers to the reproducibility of an observation. "Inter-rater reliability" refers to agreement between two or more observations of the same event at the same time (e.g., the three psychiatrists reaching the same diagnosis). "Test–retest reliability" refers to agreement between two or more observations of the event made at different times. This poses a particular problem in psychiatry because of the rapidly shifting mental status in most disorders. This chapter does not address the matter of consistency of diagnosis over time.

"Psychiatric diagnosis" is based almost exclusively on the result of the psychiatric interview, referred to by Blum (1962) as "the ultimate criterion against which other means for identifying psychiatric disorder are validated" (p. 253). At the root of our problem in psychiatric diagnostic practice is the fact that there are few antemortem or postmortem validating standards. This is explicitly acknowledged in the chapter on mental disorders in the ninth revision of the *International Classification of Diseases* (Brooke et al., 1978), wherein the inclusion of a glossary "is considered to be justified because of the special problems posed for psychiatrists by the relative lack of independent laboratory information upon which to base their diagnoses" (p. 7). "Validity" refers to the extent to which an instrument or test measures what it purports to measure. In the absence of validating data from a different body of knowledge – for example, biochemistry or pathology – proof of the validity of a diagnosis by interview cannot escape circularity. (He has schizophrenia because he has schizophrenic symptoms at interview.) This relationship between reliability and validity is summarized by Blum (1962):

To test validity one must have a criterion against which to test the accuracy of the findings achieved by the technique being examined. In psychiatric diagnosis this requirement poses a serious problem, for by definition the physician's opinion is the diagnosis and by convention, the only standard against which to test it is another physician's opinion. Such a test, if applied, is then ordinarily considered an estimate of reliability, since one is comparing two applications of the same method with one another. It is no wonder that there are but few studies which claim to escape circularity and to test the validity of the psychiatric diagnosis (p. 255).

If there is a very high degree of unreliability of the diagnostic interview for a disorder, the validity of the observations is suspect such that what is diagnosed may not exist, at least not in the sense that it approximates a definable disease entity. This is not to say that 100% reliability of observations would suddenly confer validity on a disorder, but it would be strongly suggestive. Unreliable measures are of little use even if they prove to be sporadically valid.

The field of psychiatry

"Psychiatric diagnosis" requires a little more discussion. One cannot help but be impressed by the amount of overt disagreement in the field of psychiatry over concepts of mental disease. The disagreement is far ranging and the debate often vitriolic, calling into question the actual existence of mental illness, the appropriateness of the medical model of illness, and the existence of sick patients as opposed to a sick society (Anand, 1979; Moore, 1975; Szasz, 1961). In addition, a bewildering array of models of illness have been created by the competing schools of thought, all given equal credence under the mantle of eclecticism. Although one may dismiss the extremes of the disagreement, there is no doubt that we are often faced with the need to reexamine our first principles. To use Kuhn's (1970) terminology from *The Structure of Scientific Revolutions,* psychiatry remains at the preparadigm stage in its development as a science of the mind. There is no universally accepted set of principles that define the field and define the set of problems that should and can be feasibly investigated. Thus, we cannot say that the field of psychiatry is the study and treatment of mental disorders that are caused by anatomical, biochemical, and/or physiological abnormalities of the brain. Instead, we have come to define the field, in the all-encompassing terms of the diagnostic formulators, as the study and treatment of all "abnormal" behavior caused by biological, psychological, and/or social factors. Hence, an extremely broad range of human conditions has been given the status of mental disorders. By virtue of their inclusion in the field of psychiatry, a medical specialty, they have become subject to the medical act of diagnosis. I would emphasize "medical" because the process of diagnosis is an integral part of the medical model of illness. It may not be unreasonable to suggest that for some mental disorders a medical diagnosis is nothing more than an artifact of the overinclusiveness of the field of psychiatry. This may be a major source of the reported high degree of diagnostic unreliability in psychiatry. At the very least, one must be highly suspicious of the grafting of the medical model of disease and diagnosis to the full spectrum of psychiatry as presently defined. This will become more apparent when we look at the reported differences in the degree of reliability of diagnosis for the various categories of mental disorders.

The purpose of diagnosis

It is now necessary to touch on the purposes of diagnosis that may be relevant to the topic at hand. The medical diagnosis is a shorthand description that facilitates communication among physicians. For the layman-patient, "a diagnosis is merely an intermediate step in the process of resolving the patient's complaint and is of little interest and of no intrinsic utility to the patient" (quoted by Shepherd, 1976, p. 405).

Specification of treatment

More important to the patient, a diagnosis may lead to a specific treatment. For the physician, this serves as the principal motivation to make an accurate diagnosis. If a specific remedy is not available, a diagnosis is also necessary to give an accurate prognosis to the patient and to avoid the administration of unnecessary treatment. However, the latter two reasons are only secondary to the search for a treatable cause of the patient's complaint. In the absence of specific treatment, diagnostic error is much less significant. This point is made in a report comparing autopsy findings with antemortem diagnoses (Thurlbeck, 1981). Although there was a lack of concurrence in diagnosis of the major underlying disease in 47 of 200 cases, in only 3 cases might the outcome have been affected by a correct diagnosis with different management.

The practice of psychiatry has a relatively short history of specific treatments. Electroconvulsive therapy (ECT) and psychosurgery, introduced in the late 1930s, were initially used somewhat indiscriminately, and only recently have their indications in the treatment of the more severe affective disorders become more specific. Even now over 15% of ECT is given to patients with schizophrenia, a disorder for which the indications for ECT are not well established (American Psychiatric Association, 1978). Psychotherapy has been employed much longer, but its use is ubiquitous, being applied as a remedy for almost all the mental disorders, and even very experienced practitioners have acknowledged that the nonspecific factors in the treatment may be the most essential therapeutic variables (Greben, 1977; Marmor, 1975).

Only the development of modern psychopharmaceuticals has resulted in relatively specific treatments for specific disorders. Even this statement must be qualified when one is considering the neuroleptics, which are the treatment of choice for both schizophrenia of all subtypes and severe mania. Low-dose neuroleptics have also been recommended for the treatment of so-called borderline disorders (Brinkley, Beitman, & Friedel, 1979). Although older prognostic criteria for remission of schizophrenia (Vaillant, 1964) emphasize the inclusion of features suggestive of an affective disorder, it was not until lithium carbonate was introduced as a specific prophylactic for mania that very strong emphasis was placed on the differentiation of schizophrenia from mania. Many patients previously diagnosed as schizophrenic were given trials of lithium with a successful outcome, suggesting error in the original diagnosis (Rapp & Edwards, 1977). Only recent literature has emphasized the need for more accurate diagnosis of the organic brain syndromes because some can be specifically treated and others may benefit from palliative measures (Wells, 1978).

Paradoxically, the development of a specific treatment may also lead to the overdiagnosis of the disorder for which it is specific. Psychiatrists may try to stretch the limits of the diagnosis so that many patients, otherwise considered untreatable, might at least have the benefit of a therapeutic trial of the new treatment. Notwithstanding the latter comments, it is not unreasonable to conclude that the absence of specific treatments has undermined the quest for precision in the diagnosis of certain mental disorders.

Case definition

Another main purpose of diagnosis is to indicate that the patient's complaints and mental status have exceeded the threshold for case definition. The decision as to whether the patient's symptoms and signs are clinically significant is the intuitive step that precedes consideration of a specific diagnosis: "I don't know what you've got, but whatever it is you've got a bad case of it." Blum (1962) has raised the suspicion that only a very small proportion of those who apply for psychiatric treatment are diagnosed "no illness present." These sentiments were echoed by Fleming (1981) at a trial in Ontario when he said, "There wouldn't be more than two cases a year where a psychiatrist would examine people and then call them normal." This is an important issue because it is related to the definition of the field of psychiatry previously mentioned and leads into a discussion of some of the most striking evidence of the unreliability of psychiatric diagnosis.

The reported prevalence of mental disorder in communities that have been surveyed ranges from less than 1% to greater than 80%. The Dohrenwends, in a review of the problem of validity in field studies of psychological disorder, rightly assert that "the salient question is which if any among these field studies has produced valid measures of psychological disorder" (Dohrenwend & Dohrenwend, 1965, p. 55). The wide variation in prevalence is not attributable to demographic differences in the populations surveyed. Examples of the reported high prevalence of mental disorder are of interest. In 1947, 99% of an entire Swedish community of 2,550 persons was surveyed. In 1957, Hagnell personally interviewed 99% of those still living and obtained sufficient data on others to produce a 99.6% complete survey of the original population (Hagnell, 1966). From the results of the two surveys Hagnell calculated the cumulative risk (lifetime prevalence) of developing mental illness up to age 60 years to be 44% for men and 73% for women. In Leighton's Stirling County study 31% of the sample showed a clear psychiatric disorder, another 26% showed a probable disorder, a further 26% were doubtful but still suspect of having disorder, and only 17% were considered to have no disorder (Leighton et al., 1963). The investigators concluded that at least half of the adults in Stirling County were currently suffering from some psychiatric disorder defined in the American Psychiatric Association *Diagnostic and Statistical Manual* and "at least 20% of the general population has definite need for psychiatric help, while a larger percentage would presumably be assisted by other preventive or therapeutic measures" (Leighton et al., 1963, p. 1023). Srole's survey of a sample population in Manhattan found that 23% had marked, severe, or incapacitating degrees of symptom formation, another 22% had moderate symptoms, a further 36% had mild symptoms, and only 13% were free of significant symptoms (Srole et al., 1962).

The extremely high reported prevalence of mental disorders in these examples suggests considerable difficulty in the preliminary step of case definition, let alone specific diagnosis. It is hard to take these figures seriously. Using a standardized interview and applying specific diagnostic criteria, a more recent community survey found substantially fewer "cases" – 15% of the population with a definite and 3% with a probable current diagnosis (Weissman, Myers, & Harding, 1978). Wing has also developed an index of case definition for use in community surveys (Wing et al., 1978). Based on the number, type, and severity of symptoms, the index defines a threshold point above which classification into one of the functional disorders is possible. Identification of cases using this index in the general population was highly concordant with a global clinical judgment.

Review of reliability studies

The general perception of psychiatric diagnosis is that of a very fallible exercise. In this regard, the frequently cited article "On Being Sane in Insane Places" (Rosenhan, 1973) has had an influence greatly disproportionate to its scientific merit (Spitzer, 1976). Nevertheless, the notion of ostensibly normal people being misdiagnosed as psychotic and admitted to a mental hospital is sufficiently disquieting to discredit in the minds of many the psychiatric definition of mental illness. This impression is reinforced by some of the results of early studies on diagnostic reliability. However, very important advances have been made in the standardizing of the psychiatric examination and in the development of specific diagnostic criteria for the mental disorders. If incorporated into clinical practice, these advances could lead to much greater reliability of diagnosis. It would seem likely that most of the reported literature on diagnostic reliability in psychiatry will soon be outmoded. It is for this reason that the older findings are reviewed only briefly here. As mentioned at the outset, the present discussion is concerned mainly with the more recent advances in the improvement of diagnostic reliability.

The conclusions drawn by Kreitman et al. (1961), in a review of five studies of diagnostic reliability, may be considered representative of the literature. Despite the low reliability of certain aspects of diagnosis, there is reliable differentiation of some of the major diagnostic groups. Interobserver agreement on the placement into the "generic" categories of organic brain disorder and functional psychoses is quite good (88% average for two studies in the former category and 75% in the latter). There is a marked drop in this reliability when the neuroses are considered as a group (38% for two studies). Furthermore, there was a substantial reduction in reliability for all three types of disorder when consideration changed from general to specific or four-digit diagnostic categories. Interobserver agreement on the differentiation of all diagnoses into general categories ranged between 54 and 85% but dropped to between 33 and 63% when specific diagnoses were used. The steep decline in reliability as one moves progressively from organic disorders to functional psychoses to neuroses is very evident in Kreitman's study.

Beck et al. (1962) reported an average agreement of 70% on general categories of disorder and a range of 38 to 63% agreement on specific diagnoses. Agreement on specific neurotic disorders, 63% for neurotic depressive reaction, was higher than that reported in Kreitman's review. Zubin (1967) has nicely summarized the results of many of these early studies. Once again, the progressive decline in reliability from organic disorders to functional psychoses to personality disorders and neuroses is evident.

In a study of the reasons for diagnostic disagreement, Ward et al. (1962) concluded that about one-third of the disagreements were due to variability in the interview technique and in the interpretation of the symptoms elicited. Two-thirds of the disagreements were attributed to the nosology itself – the lack of clear diagnostic criteria, the forced choice between neurotic and character disorders when both were present, and the impractically fine distinctions.

Improving diagnostic reliability

Cross-national study of diagnosis of the mental disorders

The landmark publication in this field was the April 1969 supplement to the *American Journal of Psychiatry* reporting the conceptualization and early results of the cross-national study of the diagnosis of mental disorders. The creation of the infrastructure on which more reliable diagnostic practice in psychiatry could

Table 5.1. *First-admission rates: mental hospitals,*
United States, 1957; England and Wales, 1956
(age-adjusted rates per 100,000)

Diagnosis	United States	England/Wales
All disorders	98.7	95.4
Schizophrenia	23.8	15.8
Major affective disorders	10.8	30.4
Manic–depressive	3.0	27.1
Cerebral arteriosclerosis	11.9	1.5

Source: Adapted from Kramer (1969).

be based was begun, culminating in the publication of the *Diagnostic and Statis-tical Manual of Mental Disorders* (3rd ed.) in 1980. Concluding the supplement, Heinz Lehmann (1969) wrote: "Whatever the final outcome of the study, it will almost certainly result in a sharpening and deepening of the diagnostic processes in psychiatry. This may usher in a renaissance of psychiatric diagnosis, which in many quarters today has deteriorated from being a fine and useful craft into an ill-regulated, superficial, unconvincing, and therefore often useless procedure" (p. 46).

The origins of the United States–United Kingdom diagnostic study lay in the fundamental epidemiological findings reported by Kramer (1969) in a compara-tive study of first-admission rates to mental hospitals in the United States, En-gland, and Wales. These findings are presented in abridged form in Table 5.1. It can be seen that the first-admission rates for all disorders in the United States and in England and Wales were similar. The first-admission rate for schizophre-nia in England and Wales was about one-third lower than that in the United States. The first-admission rate for manic – depressive disorder in England and Wales was nine times that in the United States. The first-admission rate for psy-chosis with cerebral arteriosclerosis in England and Wales was about one-tenth that in the United States. These figures for 1956 and 1957 were almost identical in 1960. At the time of Kramer's publication, the extent to which these figures reflected true differences in the prevalence of mental disorders was unknown.

Although a large number of variables may have contributed to these striking differences, the one that emerged as a priority for investigation was the possible difference in diagnostic practice of psychiatrists in the United States and the United Kingdom. A collaborative study evolved in which consecutive admis-sions to a mental hospital in the United States and in England were examined by a team of project psychiatrists using a standardized mental status examination. A project diagnosis was made using the eighth revision of the *Manual of the International Statistical Classification of Diseases, Injuries, and Causes of Death*

Table 5.2. *Hospital and project diagnoses: 145 consecutive admissions*

Mental disorder	Brooklyn state hospital		Netherne hospital	
	Hospital diagnosis (%)	Project diagnosis (%)	Hospital diagnosis (%)	Project diagnosis (%)
Schizophrenia	56.6	29.7	35.2	22.8
Affective disorder	16.6	36.6	46.2	58.6

Source: Adapted from Cooper et al. (1969).

(1967), and the final project diagnosis was compared with the hospital diagnosis made by the attending physician at the respective hospitals. The standardized interview used was the seventh edition of the Present State Examination developed by Wing and colleagues at the Maudsley Hospital (Wing, 1970). This instrument will be described later. The initial results of this study are summarized in Table 5.2 (Cooper et al., 1969). At the U.S. hospital, compared with hospital diagnoses there were significantly fewer project diagnoses of schizophrenia and more project diagnoses of affective illness. At the British hospital, there were also fewer project diagnoses of schizophrenia and more of affective disorder. Although the staff physicians at both hospitals tended to diagnose more schizophrenia and less affective disorder than the project psychiatrists, the tendencies were much more marked at the U.S. hospital. The very marked difference between hospitals with respect to the hospital diagnosis of schizophrenia and affective illness is substantially reduced when one compares the project diagnoses between hospitals for these disorders. A hospital diagnosis of schizophrenia was made 21% more frequently in the United States, whereas the project diagnoses reduced the difference to 7%. An affective disorder was diagnosed more than three times as frequently in the British hospital, and the project diagnosis reduced the difference to just over one and a half times. Thus, the use of a standardized interviewing technique and careful diagnostic coding according to the same classification led to a substantial reduction in the difference in the diagnoses between the two countries.

That these differences in hospital admission statistics reflected cross-national differences in the conceptualization of mental disorders is quite clearly demonstrated by the studies of Katz, Cole, and Lowery (1969) and Copeland et al. (1971). Rating a videotape interview of the same patient, one-third of the American psychiatrists diagnosed schizophrenia, whereas none of the British psychiatrists made that diagnosis. About one-third of the Americans diagnosed personality disorder, whereas 59% of the British made that diagnosis.

The apparent overdiagnosis of schizophrenia in the United States is clearly related to the very broad concept of the disorder held by many American psychiatrists. The concept of "pseudoneurotic schizophrenia" introduced by Hoch and Polatin in 1949 carried undue influence. Perhaps representative of this broad concept of the disorder are the comments of Nolan Lewis, a former director of the New York State Psychiatric Institute, that, as in the diagnosis of pregnancy, "even a trace of schizophrenia is schizophrenia" (quoted by Kuriansky et al., 1977, p. 635).

Standardized clinical examination

How can appropriate concepts of mental disorders be reached? The psychiatric literature contains numerous references to the pressing need for increased standardization of the psychiatric examination (Feinstein, 1977). Indeed, the cornerstone of the American – British comparative study was the use of a standardized clinical interview. At this point, it would be useful to give some idea of the complexity of developing such standardization given the present state of the art of psychiatry. The Present State Examination (PSE) was developed by the Medical Research Council social psychiatry unit in London under the direction of Professor J. Wing (Wing, 1970). The PSE was developed for purposes of reliably describing cases for the international pilot study of schizophrenia for the World Health Organization. It has had numerous modifications during its development and has reached a ninth edition. A very high inter-rater reliability has been achieved with this instrument (Wing et al., 1967). The schedule is designed to elicit in a standardized way the presence of any symptoms of psychiatric disorder present in the 1 month preceding the interview as well as a rating of abnormal behavior present during the interview.

The importance of the standardization lies in its precise definition of symptoms and signs and its completeness. In order to be rated, a symptom must be present in a form and degree sufficient to meet threshold criteria. The schedule was designed with sufficiently high symptom thresholds to avoid ratings that might represent only minor deviations from the normal. The intent was to minimize the frequency of false positive ratings. In keeping with good clinical practice, many of the ratings require an example of the patient's response to be written on the coding sheet. Unlike a simple questionnaire in which clarification of the items may not be given, the interpretation of the items is not left to the patient such that a yes or no reply is insufficient to make a rating. Once again, the intent was to eliminate false positives through exclusion of the normal angst, ennui, and dysphoria of the human condition.

As previously noted, the PSE was designed primarily as an instrument to standardize the description of psychiatric syndromes, particularly schizophrenia, for purposes of international epidemiological studies. Recognizing the deficiencies of the current psychiatric nomenclature, the instrument was not designed to yield current *International Classification of Diseases* diagnoses. However, the phenomenological basis for the instrument does conform to certain current concepts of the major psychiatric syndromes, and therefore the instrument yields descriptive data that can readily be grouped into classes closely resembling conventional diagnostic groups. Emanating from the Maudsley school, the emphasis lies on the Schneiderian concept of schizophrenia. Although not universally accepted as the diagnostic criteria of choice and certainly not considered necessary criteria for many patients who would be called schizophrenic by most clinicians, the Schneiderian first-rank symptoms are perhaps more clearly definable and more reliably rated than many of the Bleulerian symptoms. As implied by their designation as first rank, the presence of one or more of the symptoms in this group has been considered to be almost pathognomonic of schizophrenia. The corollary is that the absence of first-rank symptoms decreases the likelihood of schizophrenia being the correct diagnosis. Unfortunately, the diagnostic significance of such a finding is not so clear-cut. At present, it is more appropriate to state that there is no single pathognomonic symptom or sign of schizophrenia, the presence or absence of which confirms or refutes the diagnosis. We simply do not know how many patients who have schizophrenia, whatever that may prove to be, do have Schneiderian symptoms at some point in the course of their illness and how many never experience such symptoms. In addition, if the first-rank symptoms are not pathognomonic of schizophrenia, they may well occur in the course of any number of other syndromes, and the frequency of such occurrences is also unknown (Carpenter, Strauss, & Mulek, 1973; Mellor, 1970; Taylor, 1972).

Thus, at present we are faced with unknown probabilities of the presence or absence of any given symptom in any given patient with the syndrome schizophrenia. In addition, there is no clear correlation between any given symptom and any particular course of illness.

An alternative to considering the Schneiderian symptoms pathognomonic of schizophrenia is to place them at the top of a hierarchy of symptoms, ranked according to the probability or certainty of their being part of the syndrome "schizophrenia." The PSE places the Schneiderian first-rank symptoms at the top of such a hierarchy. Thus, rather than making unwarranted assumptions about which symptoms are pathognomonic of a syndrome that to date is definable only by symptoms, this method approaches the problem of conceptualizing a syndrome through a series of probability statements, something along the following line. The presence of symptom X increases the probability of the patient having schizophrenia, whatever schizophrenia may prove to be. The absence of symptom X decreases that probability. The presence of symptom X increases the probability of symptoms Y and Z being present. The absence of symptom X decreases that probability. The presence of symptoms Y and Z in combination with symptom X further increases the probability of the presence of the syndrome "schizophrenia.'' This is the series of steps used in the design of programs for diagnosing medical disorders wherein data from the history, physical examination, and laboratory tests are fed into a computer. The only difference in psychiatric syndromes is the absence of any validating data. Of course, this remains a somewhat circular process but not quite as circular as the clinical impression that the patient is schizophrenic because he has schizophrenic symptoms.

The PSE groups symptoms into a number of syndromes. Symptoms considered most likely to be part of the syndrome ''schizophrenia'' are grouped together into the so-called nuclear syndrome, which is sufficient by itself to place a patient in the major class designated S +. Patients are considered to have nuclear schizophrenia. No other single PSE syndrome is sufficient alone to place a patient in the S + class, suggesting that the authors of the PSE do tend to consider these symptoms pathognomonic of at least one type of schizophrenia. The other PSE syndromes are placed in a hierarchy according to their probability of being diagnostic of a particular disorder or their weighting in support of a diagnosis in combination with one or more other syndromes. Those PSE syndromes that normally would be considered by themselves suggestive of a diagnosis of affective psychosis are used to support the decision to place the patient in a schizophrenic or paranoid psychosis class when they occur in combination with any of a number of delusional syndromes. Thus, PSE symptoms and syndromes are hierarchically ranked and weighted both according to their probability of forming part of a particular diagnostic syndrome and according to a sequence of diagnostic syndromes that gives priority to the schizophrenic, paranoid, and borderline psychoses over the affective and neurotic syndromes.

The authors of the PSE have developed a computer program designed to group the symptom ratings according to clinically relevant clusters that yield successive approximations of the conventional nosology. In effect, the program replicates the clinical decision-making process according to the authors' notion of the diagnostic criteria for the various psychiatric syndromes. The use of a computer program simply ensures that the presence of a specific combination of PSE ratings will always result in placement in the same group (Wing, Cooper, & Sartorius, 1974).

At this point, it is again well to remember that the PSE and its computerized analysis were founded on the current concepts of phenomenology and nosology even though these concepts are considered inadequate. The developers of the instrument recognized this limitation and defined it only as a means to yield uniform descriptions of patients for epidemiological studies. The successive approximations to ICD diagnoses simply provide a variety of descriptions varying in detail for comparative purposes.

The standardized interview schedules exemplified by the PSE are very lengthy and their analysis very complex. Therefore, they have not found widespread acceptance in clinical practice. Revisions of the classification system appear to offer more immediate promise for the improvement of diagnostic reliability.

Progress in psychiatric nosology: DSM III

As mentioned earlier, a major source of the diagnostic unreliability previously reported has been the diagnostic classification itself. The failure to provide explicit inclusion and exclusion criteria and the need to make forced choices between syndromes with considerable conceptual overlap has certainly been a deficiency equal to the lack of standardized examination techniques. The American classification has gone a long way toward eliminating these deficiencies.

The *Diagnostic and Statistical Manual of Mental Disorders,* third edition (DSM III) (1980), was developed by the American Psychiatric Association Task Force on Nomenclature and Statistics, chaired by Robert Spitzer. The DSM has a short history; the first edition, published in 1952, was followed by a second edition in 1968 based on the concurrently published eighth revision of the ICD. The American isolationists have regained ascendancy as DSM III parts company with its World Health Organization counterpart, ICD-9. The four-digit codes of ICD-9 were expanded to codes of five digits, including many of the developing DSM III categories, and in 1979 this ICD-9-CM (clinical modification) became the official system for recording morbidity and mortality statistics in the United States.

Diagnostic criteria. The conceptualization of the DSM III format was continuous with that of the Research Diagnostic Criteria (RDC) developed by Spitzer's group as part of a collaborative project on the depressive disorders sponsored by the National Institute of Mental Health (Endicott & Spitzer, 1978; Spitzer, Endicott, & Robins, 1978). In turn, the RDC began as a modification of the 1972 "Feighner criteria" of the St. Louis group (Feighner et al., 1972). The objective of this work has been the definition of reliable diagnostic criteria for distinct and homogeneous clinical disorders to be used in sample selection for research purposes. Unfortunately, the application of rigid research criteria to a ward full of patients may suddenly "cure" them all because they no longer fulfill the criteria for the disorders for which they are being treated. In deference to the principal goal of a clinically useful classification, some of the criteria have been relaxed in DSM III. Nevertheless, this quest for improved diagnostic reliability and homogeneity through the inclusion of specific diagnostic criteria for each disorder represents the most useful contribution of DSM III (Spitzer, Williams, & Skodol, 1980).

Multiaxial classification. The multiaxial concept was borrowed from that reported by Rutter, Shaffer, and Shepherd (1975) for childhood disorders. This triaxial classification included the clinical syndrome, intellectual level, and etiological factors. The multiaxial system of DSM III simply formalized the recording of multiple diagnoses and certain nondiagnostic descriptive data considered useful in planning treatment and predicting outcome. Axis I includes most of the clinical syndromes and a group of conditions not attributable to a mental disorder that are a focus of attention or treatment. The personality disorders and specific developmental or learning disorders are relegated to Axis II with the assurance that this is not to imply that these are not mental disorders but rather to ensure that they are not overlooked in the presence of a more florid Axis I disorder. This addresses the previously mentioned criticism of the nosology that required a forced choice between coexistent personality disorder and another syndrome. The third axis for physical disorders completes the official diagnostic assessment. Axis IV, severity of psychosocial stressors, and Axis V, highest level of adaptive functioning in the past year, are optional, and the text describes rather simplistic ratings for each.

In the following paragraphs, a few of the major changes in the conceptualization of the mental disorders as presented in DSM III and some of the diagnostic criteria are reviewed.

Schizophrenia. The subtyping of schizophrenia has been substantially revised, and the diagnostic criteria for schizophrenia of any kind require the presence of psychotic features at some time in the course of illness. Therefore, the subtype of simple schizophrenia, often used in the absence of florid symptoms, has been completely deleted and replaced by an approximation under the personality disorders (schizotypal personality disorder). Similarly, latent schizophrenia is replaced by borderline personality disorder. The diagnostic criterion of a 6-month duration automatically excludes acute schizophrenic episodes, such cases to be included in the schizophreniform, brief reactive psychosis, or schizoaffective disorder categories. Schneiderian first-rank symptoms are given prominence. Although less florid prodromal or residual symptoms may have been present during the 6-month period, that interval must also include an active phase of illness in which at least one of the symptoms from the first diagnostic criterion was present.

Affective disorders. The affective disorders have been grouped together in recognition of the constraints imposed by dichotomizing the group with one variable (psychotic–nonpsychotic, endogenous–reactive). Thus, the presence or absence of psychotic symptoms is not a primary determinant of diagnosis and is only appended to other diagnoses (i.e., major depression with psychotic features). The bipolar–unipolar concept has been adopted as the principal basis for subtyping the major affective disorders into bipolar disorder and major depression.

Involutional melancholia involutes and disappears as a distinct entity with the rationale that depression occurring in the involutional period is indistinguishable from that occurring at other times.

Neuroses. The term "neurosis" has gone the way of the "vapors" in DSM III. The frequently used term has come to mean much more than the classical symptom neuroses. In addition to its descriptive use, the term also implies a theoretical etiological process. In keeping with its atheoretical approach, DSM III abolishes the term and groups the "neurotic" disorders in a number of categories each of which has a generic symptom or group of symptoms as the basis for classification rather than the theoretical etiology.

Depressive neurosis is subsumed under major depression (without psychotic features or melancholia), dysthymic disorder, or adjustment disorder with depressed mood. Identifiable events considered to be of etiological significance can be coded on Axis IV. Phobic neurosis has become a group of disorders (agoraphobia with or without panic attacks, social and simple phobia, and separation anxiety disorder of childhood). Anxiety neurosis has been divided into panic disorder and generalized anxiety disorder. The obsessive compulsive neurosis has simply changed from neurosis to disorder. Hysterical neurosis has been classified under the somatoform (conversion and psychogenic pain disorders) and dissociative disorders (psychogenic amnesia and fugue, multiple personality, and sleepwalking). Neurasthenic neurosis has been dropped, because the malign effects of masturbation no longer include this syndrome.

Psychosexual disorders. The sexual disorders are no longer subsumed under sexual deviations but are grouped and more completely enumerated under gender identity disorders, paraphilias, and other disorders. A new category of psychosexual dysfunctions has been added to include those who seek psychiatric help in their quest for the complete orgasm. The longest and most detailed explanatory note for a change in the classification is that for homosexuality to egodystonic homosexuality. In spite of the explanation, there is no doubt that this change, preceded in 1973 by sexual orientation disturbance, was almost entirely in response to a strong homosexual lobby rather than any advance in knowledge (Stoller et al., 1973).

Antisocial personality disorder. Of particular interest to readers of this volume will be the diagnostic criteria for the antisocial personality disorder presented in Table 5.3 in an abridged form. It can be seen that the criteria are almost exclusively descriptive of behavior. Examination for the presence or absence of these criteria does not require an interview with the patient except to exclude the presence of other disorders. This strong emphasis on purely behavioral criteria is

Table 5.3. *DSM III diagnostic criteria for antisocial personality disorder*

A. Current age at least 18
B. Onset before age 15, as indicated by a history, of three or more of the following:
    1. Truancy (at least 5 days per year for at least 2 years, not including the last year of school)
    2. Expulsion or suspension from school
    3. Delinquency (arrested or referred to juvenile court)
    4. Running away from home overnight at least twice
    5. Persistent lying
    6. Repeated sexual intercourse in a casual relationship
    7. Repeated drunkenness or substance abuse
    8. Thefts
    9. Vandalism
    10. School grades markedly below expectations for IQ
    11. Chronic violations of rules at home and/or at school
    12. Initiation of fights
C. At least four of the following since age 18:
    1. Inability to sustain consistent work behavior
    2. Lack of ability to function as a responsible parent
    3. Failure to accept social norms with respect to lawful behavior
    4. Inability to maintain enduring attachment to a sexual partner
    5. Irritability and aggressiveness as indicated by repeated physical fights or assault
    6. Failure to honor financial obligations
    7. Failure to plan ahead or impulsivity
    8. Recklessness, as indicated by driving while intoxicated or recurrent speeding
D. Pattern of continuous antisocial behavior in which the rights of others are violated, with no intervening period of at least 5 years without antisocial behavior between age 15 and the present time (except when the individual was bedridden or confined in a hospital or penal institution)
E. Pattern of antisocial behavior that is not due to severe mental retardation, schizophrenia, or manic episodes

related to the earlier reference to the prediction of behavior. The global term ''antisocial personality'' is of much less predictive usefulness than is the precise itemization of the antisocial behaviors and their temporal sequence to determine whether there has been progressive escalation of severity or whether a particular behavior is a sporadic or isolated event.

Social definition of disease. At this point a comment on the overall validity of the psychiatric nomenclature may be in order. Only in psychiatry could we have a published symposium entitled ''Changing Styles in Psychiatric Syndromes'' (Schimel et al., 1973). The validity of the psychiatric nosology is definitely affected by the role of social forces in shaping mental disorders, both in defining behavior that is considered deviant and in determining the symptomatic expression of that deviance. On the evolutionary time scale, societies and their mores change much faster than human anatomy and physiology such that socially defined disorders may come and go, leading one to question the whole process

Table 5.4. *DSM III diagnostic criteria for dementia*

A. Loss of intellectual abilities of sufficient severity to interfere with social or occupational functioning
B. Memory impairment
C. At least one of the following:
   1. Impairment of abstract thinking
   2. Impaired judgment
   3. Other disturbances of higher cortical function, such as aphasia, apraxia, agnosia, "constructional difficulty"
   4. Personality change
D. State of consciousness not clouded (i.e., criteria for delirium or intoxication not met, although these may be superimposed)
E. Either of the following:
   1. Evidence from the history, physical examination, or laboratory tests of a specific organic factor that is judged to be etiologically related to the disturbance
   2. In the absence of such evidence, the presumption of an organic factor necessary for the development of the syndrome if conditions other than organic mental disorders have been reasonably excluded *and if the behavioral change represents cognitive impairment in a variety of areas*

---

whereby disorders can be created and "cured" by ephemeral moral suasion. Thus, onanism becomes narcissism, homosexuality becomes normal in deference to a political lobby, neurosis disappears, in part a result of a move away from the Victorian notion of repressed sexuality as a unifying concept for a group of disorders, and Russian psychiatrists gerrymander their nosology to serve nefarious political purposes (Reich, 1975).

Clinical practice and diagnostic criteria

Having described the DSM III diagnostic criteria, we can now look at them in relation to some actual clinical practice. For this purpose we shall select a disorder in which the presence or absence of the diagnostic criteria should be relatively easy to document, that is, primary degenerative dementia, or Alzheimer's disease. This may not seem to be particularly relevant to the theme of this book, but the example does highlight some of the problems with current psychiatric practice in relation to the use of diagnostic criteria. Table 5.4 presents the diagnostic criteria for primary degenerative dementia. Table 5.5 shows the frequency with which the various areas of cognitive function were examined in 63 patients given a discharge diagnosis of dementia at the Clarke Institute of Psychiatry between 1974 and 1979. The area was considered to have been examined, however incompletely, if any one test of that function was performed or if the medical record inferred that the area had been examined at all. Although memory, orientation, judgment, and insight were examined in almost all cases, what should

Table 5.5. *Examination of cognitive function in demented patients*

Cognitive function	Not examined[a]	Uncooperative; not examined	Examined	Response recorded
Memory				
Recent	4 (6)	1	58	48
Remote	4 (6)	1	58	42
Orientation				
Person	10 (16)	0	53	23
Place	5 (8)	0	58	27
Time	1 (2)	0	62	35
Concentration	13 (21)	3	47	28
General knowledge	30 (48)	3	30	23
Abstraction	31 (49)	5	27	9
Calculation	39 (62)	3	21	10
Aphasia	54 (86)	0	9	6
Agnosia	57 (90)	0	6	2
Apraxia	51 (81)	0	12	10
Judgment	9 (14)	1	53	32
Insight	6 (10)	0	57	33

[a] Nearest whole percentage in parentheses.

be noted is the remarkably low frequency with which the other areas of cognitive function were examined. Testing of aphasia, agnosia, and apraxia, including constructional apraxia, was done in very few cases, and yet impairment in these areas is one of the diagnostic criteria for dementia. The other diagnostic criterion of note is that of progressive deterioration in cognitive function for Alzheimer's disease. A follow-up examination to document that deterioration was not performed in over 85% of these cases (Martin, Peter, & Eastwood, 1983).

Conclusion

We are so very far from understanding the pathophysiology of the mental disorders. Despite substantive advances in the fields of genetics, biochemistry, and pharmacology, the models of illness derived therefrom have been inadequate to explain all the data, and the treatments based on those models have been only qualified successes. Even in the case of the affective disorders in which conceptual advances have appeared to be very significant, identification of the biological substrate of the disorders remains elusive (Lehmann, 1977). The recent hypothesis of a kindling model for mania and its prophylaxis with carbamazepine

(Tegretol), a treatment of choice for temporal lobe epilepsy, seems to be a great distance from the catecholamine hypothesis and its derivatives (Ballenger & Post, 1980; Post & Kapanda, 1976). Moreover, we do not have a single diagnostic test for any of the "functional" disorders.

It might be wise to remain skeptical of the prediction in an issue of *Schizophrenia Bulletin* that DSM IV may include specific biological tests to define affective disorders and that the DSM V may include similar tests for schizophrenia (Haier, 1980). As far as the clinical practice of psychiatry is concerned, we remain dependent on our observations at interview to create order out of our patients' complaints and on our classification system to create order out of our observations.

Naming, counting, and classification have absorbed the obsessional among us since Linnaeus (1707–78) began to create order in apparently diverse biological systems with his binomial nomenclature of genera and species. The variegated symptoms and signs of human illnesses began to coalesce into specific diseases under Thomas Sydenham's (1624–39) careful observation of their natural history. Emil Kraepelin made the first major contribution to the science of nosology in psychiatry, once again through observation of the natural history of disease, separating the unremitting course of dementia praecox from that of manic–depressive psychosis. In clinical practice, we have not outgrown this need for careful observation and description. We remain largely at the syndrome stage in psychiatry, with specific diseases yet to be described. Schizophrenia is analogous to the "fevers." Whether the description will come from the laboratory or the bedside remains to be seen.

What I have discussed here is not at the cutting edge of psychiatric research. It is more fundamental. Reliable clinical observations of symptoms and signs leading to reliable diagnosis is the sine qua non of clinical research. The operative word here is "research." To borrow Freud's metaphor, the royal road to reliability is not through dreaming but through the hard work of developing standardized clinical observations and better classifications of those observations. As discussed in this chapter, both of these monumental undertakings have been the product of research endeavors.

But what about clinical practice? To put it as gently as possible, something is lost in the translation from research to clinical practice. Strupp (1960) nicely articulated the isolation of research from clinical practice in his paper "Some Comments on the Future of Research in Psychotherapy": "I believe that up to the present, research contributions have had exceedingly little influence on the practical procedures of psychotherapy" (p. 63). More closely related to the items of this book is the footnote of Bartholemew and Milte (1976): "More recent work shows that when special steps are taken to avoid the most obvious sources of inter-observer variation, for instance by using standardized interview schedules and agreed glossaries of diagnostic terms, satisfactory levels of reliability and repeatability of the various stages of the diagnostic process can be achieved. This may be true for a specific research endeavor but reliability remains poor in routine clinical work, including the opinions offered in court by forensic psychiatrists'' (p. 452).

In conclusion, we have the wherewithal to improve diagnostic reliability in psychiatric practice. However, one might ask whether the degree of regimentation imposed by both standardized clinical interviews and the DSM III diagnostic criteria is anathema to most psychiatrists. If so, their widespread introduction into clinical practice will be a long time coming.

References

Anand, R. Involuntary civil commitment in Ontario: The need to curtail the abuses of psychiatry. *Canadian Bar Review,* 1979, *57,* 250–80.

Ballenger, J. C., & Post, R. M. Carbamazepine in manic – depressive illness: A new treatment. *American Journal of Psychiatry,* 1980, *137,* 782–90.

Bartholomew, A. A., & Milte, K. L. The reliability and validity of psychiatric diagnoses in courts of law. *Australia Law Journal,* 1976, *50,* 450–8.

Beck, A. T., Ward, C. H., Mendelson, M., Mock, J. E., & Erbaugh, J. K. Reliability of psychiatric diagnoses. 2. A Study of consistency of clinical judgments and ratings. *American Journal of Psychiatry,* 1962, *119,* 351–7.

Blum, R. H. Case identification in psychiatric epidemiology: Methods and problems. *Millbank Memorial Fund Quarterly,* 1962, *40,* 253–88.

Brinkley, J. R., Beitman, B. D., & Friedel, R. O. Low-dose neuroleptic regimens in the treatment of borderline patients. *Archives of General Psychiatry,* 1979, *36,* 319–26.

Brooke, E. M., Cooper, J. E., Jablensky, A., Kramer, M., & Sartorius, N. *Mental disorders: Glossary and guide to their classification in accordance with the ninth revision of the international classification of diseases.* Geneva: World Health Organization, 1978.

Carpenter, W. T., Strauss, J. S., & Mulek, S. Are there pathognomonic symptoms in schizophrenia? An empiric investigation of Schneider's first-rank symptoms. *Archives of General Psychiatry,* 1973, *28,* 847–52.

Cooper, J. E., Kendell, R. E., Gurland, B. J., Sartorius, N., & Farkas, T. Cross-national study of diagnosis of the mental disorders: Some results from the first comparative investigation. *American Journal of Psychiatry,* 1969, *125,* 21–9.

Copeland, J. R. M., Cooper, J. E., Kendell, R. E., & Gourlay, A. J. Differences in usage of diagnostic labels amongst psychiatrists in the British Isles. *British Journal of Psychiatry,* 1971, *118,* 629–40.

Diagnostic and statistical manual of mental disorders (3rd ed.). Washington, D.C.: American Psychiatric Association, 1980.

Dohrenwend, B. P., & Dohrenwend, B. S. The problem of validity in field studies of psychological disorder. *Journal of Abnormal Psychology,* 1965, *70,* 52–69.

Endicott, J., & Spitzer, R. L. A diagnostic interview: The schedule for affective disorders and schizophrenia. *Archives of General Psychiatry,* 1978, *35,* 837–44.

Feighner, J. P., Robins, E., Guze, S. B., Woodruff, R. A., Winokur, G., & Munoz, R. Diagnostic criteria for use in psychiatric research. *Archives of General Psychiatry,* 1972, *26,* 57–63.

Feinstein, A. R. A critical overview of diagnosis in psychiatry. In V. M. Rakoff, H. C. Stancer, & H. B. Kedward (Eds.), *Psychiatric diagnosis.* New York: Brunner Mazel, 1977.

Fleming, R. Quoted in the *Toronto Star, December 2, 1981.

Greben, S. E. On being therapeutic. *Canadian Psychiatric Association Journal,* 1977, *22,* 371–80.

Hagnell, O. *A Prospective Study of the Incidence of Mental Disorder.* Stockholm: Svenska Bokforlaget, 1966.

Haier, R. J. The diagnosis of schizophrenia: A review of recent developments. *Schizophrenia Bulletin,* 1980, *6,* 417–28.

Hoch, P., & Polatin, P. Pseudoneurotic forms of schizophrenia. *Psychiatry Quarterly,* 1949, *23,* 248–76.

Katz, M. M., Cole, J. O., & Lowery, H. A. Studies of the diagnostic process: The influence of symptom perception, past experience, and ethnic background on diagnostic decisions. *American Journal of Psychiatry,* 1969, *125,* 937–47.

Kramer, M. Cross-national study of diagnosis of the mental disorders: Origin of the problem. *American Journal of Psychiatry,* 1969, *125,* 1–11.

Kreitman, N., Sainsbury, P., Morrissey, J., Towers, J., and Scrivener, J. The reliability of psychiatric assessment: An analysis. *Journal of Mental Science,* 1961, *107,* 887–908.

Kuhn, T. S. *The structure of scientific revolutions.* Chicago: University of Chicago Press, 1970.

Kuriansky, J. B., Gurland, B. J., Spitzer, R. L., & Endicott, J. Trends in the frequency of schizophrenia by different diagnostic criteria. *American Journal of Psychiatry,* 1977, *134,* 631–6.

Lehmann, H. E. A renaissance of psychiatric diagnosis? *American Journal of Psychiatry,* 1969, *125,* 43–6.

Lehmann, H. E. Classification of depressive states. *Canadian Psychiatric Association Journal,* 1977, *22,* 381–90.

Leighton, D. C., Harding, J. S., Macklin, D. B., Hughes, C. C., & Leighton, A. H. Psychiatric findings of the Stirling County study. *American Journal of Psychiatry,* 1963, *119,* 1021–6.

Lipkin, M. The CPC as an anachronism. *New England Journal of Medicine,* 1979, *301,* 1113–14.

Manual of the international statistical classification of diseases, injuries, and causes of death (8th rev. ed). Geneva: World Health Organization, 1967.

Marmor, J. The nature of the psychotherapeutic process revisited. *Canadian Psychiatric Association Journal,* 1975, *20,* 557–65.

Martin, B. A., Peter, A. M., & Eastwood, M. R. The mental status examination for dementia: A review of practice in a psychiatric hospital. *Canadian Journal of Psychiatry,* 1983, *28,* 287–90.

Mellor, C. S. First rank symptoms in schizophrenia. 1. The frequency in schizophrenics on admission to hospital. 2. Differences between individual first rank symptoms. *British Journal of Psychiatry,* 1970, *117,* 15–23.

Moore, M. S. Some myths about "mental illness." *Archives of General Psychiatry,* 1975, *32,* 1483–97.

Post, R. M., & Kapanda, R. T. Cocaine, kindling and psychosis. *American Journal of Psychiatry,* 1976, *133,* 627–34.

Rapp, M. S., & Edwards, P. A high prevalence of affective disorder discovered in a "schizophrenic clinic." *Canadian Psychiatric Association Journal,* 1977, *22,* 181–3.

Reich, W. The spectrum concept of schizophrenia. *Archives of General Psychiatry,* 1975, *32,* 489–98.

Rosenhan, D. L. On being sane in insane places. *Science,* 1973, *179,* 250–8.

Rutter, M., Shaffer, D., & Shepherd, M. *A multi-axial classification of child psychiatric disorders.* Geneva: World Health Organization, 1975.

Schimel, J. L., Salzman, L., Chodoff, P., Grinker, R. R., & Will, O. A. Changing styles in psychiatric syndromes: A symposium. *American Journal of Psychiatry,* 1973, *130,* 146–55.

Scully, R. E. In defense of the CPC. *New England Journal of Medicine,* 1979, *301,* 1114–16.

Shepherd, M. The extent of mental disorder: Beyond the layman's madness. *Canadian Psychiatric Association Journal,* 1976, *21,* 401–9.

Spitzer, R. L. More on pseudoscience in science and the case for psychiatric diagnosis. *Archives of General Psychiatry*, 1976, *33*, 459–70.

Spitzer, R. L., Endicott, J., & Robins, E. Research diagnostic criteria: Rationale and reliability. *Archives of General Psychiatry*, 1978, *35*, 773–82.

Spitzer, R. L., Williams, J. B. W., & Skodol, A. E. DSM-III: The major achievements and an overview. *American Journal of Psychiatry*, 1980, *137*, 151–64.

Srole, L., Langner, T. S., Michael, S. T., Opler, M. K., & Rennie, T. A. C. *Mental health in the metropolis: The Midtown Manhattan Study*, (Vol. 1). New York: McGraw-Hill, 1962.

Stoller, R. J., Marmor, J., Bieber, I., Gold, R., Socarides, C. W., Green, R., & Spitzer, R. L. A symposium: Should homosexuality be in the APA nomenclature? *American Journal of Psychiatry*, 1973, *130*, 1207–16.

Strupp, H. H. Some comments on the future of research in psychotherapy. *Behavioural Science*, 1960, *5*, 60–71.

Szasz, T. S. *The myth of mental illness*. New York: Dell, 1961.

Task force report 14: Electroconvulsive therapy. Washington, D.C.: American Psychiatric Association, 1978.

Taylor, M. A. Schneiderian first-rank symptoms and clinical prognostic features in schizophrenia. *Archives of General Psychiatry*, 1972, *26*, 64–7.

Thurlbeck, W. M. Accuracy of clinical diagnosis in a Canadian teaching hospital. *Canadian Medical Association Journal*, 1981, *125*, 443–7.

Vaillant, G. E. Prospective prediction of schizophrenic remission. *Archives of General Psychiatry*, 1964, *2*, 509–18.

Ward, C. H., Beck, A. T., Mendelson, M., Mock, J. E., & Erbaugh, J. K. The psychiatric nomenclature: Reasons for diagnostic disagreement. *Archives of General Psychiatry*, 1962, *7*, 198–205.

Weissman, M. M., Myers, J. K., & Harding, P. S. Psychiatric disorders in a U.S. urban community: 1975–1976. *American Journal of Psychiatry*, 1978, *135*, 459–62.

Wells, C. E. Chronic brain disease: An overview. *American Journal of Psychiatry*, 1978, *135*, 1–12.

Wing, J. K. A standard form of psychiatric Present State Examination. In E. H. Hare & J. K. Wing (Eds.), *Psychiatric epidemiology*. London: Nuffield Prov. Hospital Trust, Oxford University Press, 1970.

Wing, J. K., Birley, J. L. T., Cooper, J. E., Graham, P., & Isaacs, A. D. Reliability of a procedure for measuring and classifying "present psychiatric state." *British Journal of Psychiatry*, 1967, *113*, 499–515.

Wing, J. K., Cooper, J. E., & Sartorius, N. *The measurement and classification of psychiatric symptoms*. Cambridge: Cambridge University Press, 1974.

Wing, J. K., Mann, S. A., Leff, J. P., & Nixon, J. M. The concept of a "case" in psychiatric population surveys. *Psychological Medicine*, 1978, *8*, 203–17.

Zubin, J. Classification of the behavior disorders. *Annual Review of Psychology*, 1967, *18*, 373–406.

6   Hypothetical criteria for the prediction of individual criminality

Park Elliott Dietz

This chapter, it should be said at the outset, is a theoretical essay, not a review or a research report. It defines a residual class of "intolerable crimes"[1] for which it might be reasonable to expect clinicians to attempt predictive judgments for the purpose of preventing harm to potential victims. It also outlines the sources of information to be garnered in rendering such predictions and hypothesizes first-, second-, and third-rank predictors grouped according to their predictive weights.

The purpose and scope of prediction

Individual crime prediction by clinicians has three purposes: (a) injury control, that is, the protection of potential victims; (b) paternalism, that is, the protection of the individual from the consequences of his or her potential criminal actions; and (c) self-protection, that is, the elimination of personal responsibility (and legal liability) of the clinician for the deleterious consequences of negligent predictive errors. This chapter concerns only the first of these,[2] for the protection of potential victims is the basis for the social-control functions of forensic medicine and clinical criminology. It is assumed here that the circumstances of prediction are those in which clinicians assist legitimate authority in deciding whether to incapacitate an individual through a lengthy confinement to protect potential victims.[3]

Monahan (1981) has written that progress in prediction requires "a dramatic increase in the degree to which mental health professionals articulate what it is they are predicting and how they went about predicting it" (p. 17). In this section, an effort is made to articulate the former; in a later section, a strategy is proposed for conceptualizing the latter.

We are, of course, not interested in predicting just any crime, because that task is too simple: We may predict with reasonable certainty that any individual before us will at some future time engage in some criminal act, because a large proportion of the general population will do so. It is therefore not all criminal

87

acts that we mean to predict but only certain types.[4] The crimes focused on here are a small but important subset of all crimes called "intolerable," but not all are intolerable in the same way. Some are intolerable because of their gravity or the number of victims, some because of their impact on society as a whole, and some because they are perceived to be both serious and predictable.[5] Serious crimes that are intolerable because they are perceived to be predictable are those committed by individuals who had previously come to clinical, judicial, or correctional attention and who were known to have made threats or to have evidenced behavior that is widely viewed as dangerous.[6]

Violent and otherwise dangerous crimes that occur with high frequency, such as murder, battery, forcible rape, armed robbery, arson, burglary, and drunk and reckless driving, could be reduced by certain environmental countermeasures, such as those related to firearms, building security, and passenger protection systems. However, the widespread public acceptance, at least in the United States, of the excessive consumption of alcohol, private possession of firearms, and irresponsible design and use of motor vehicles suggests that the public regards a substantial amount of murder, armed robbery, and destruction with motor vehicles as tolerable costs of highly prized liberties.[7] The means by which the public may decrease the incidence and severity of injuries from these behaviors are already within reach of public officials, who are better equipped than clinicians to implement them.

Certain other intolerable crimes that are quite infrequent, such as assassination, terrorist acts, and skyjacking, can also be reduced more through other means than through clinical prediction. Examples of preferred countermeasures include a decrease in the frequency of public appearances of political figures for the prevention of assassination, domestic surveillance activities for the prevention of terrorist acts, and screening of airline passengers for metallic materials for the prevention of skyjacking. Like clinical prediction, nonclinical countermeasures have costs that policy makers must weigh against benefits, but the clinician's role in policy debates over security versus liberty should usually be that of an advocate for security for his or her patients and for others.

If these other classes of criminal behavior were put aside because of the availability of higher-priority preventive strategies, the types of intolerable crimes left for clinicians to worry about would be few. They would include sadistic sexual assaults and murders, serial murders of all kinds, bombings, arson, and intrafamilial violence. As it happens, these are precisely the offenses that are most predictable. As illustrated later, however, they are predictable only because individuals who commit them often do so repetitively, allowing one to predict subsequent offenses only after at least one offense has been threatened or completed.

To this group of intolerable crimes we must add all other murders, batteries, and rapes occurring after a clinical evaluation of "dangerousness" that elicited information that a reasonably prudent clinician would regard as predictive of future violence. We must do so not only for the obvious paternalistic and self-protective reasons, but also because society has delegated to us (and to others, such as law enforcement officers) the responsibility of making judgments of "dangerousness" among those who come to our attention in our professional capacities. Although many clinicians eschew this policemanlike role, I think we have a moral duty to the potential victims of those whom we evaluate. Like the legal duty that has been recognized in some jurisdictions, this moral duty does not require perfect prediction, only reasonable prudence in the exercise of professional judgment.

Sources of information

The most remediable error in the clinical prediction of crime is the making of a prediction without sufficient data to provide a basis for informed judgment. The lack of sufficient data most often reflects resource constraints. The vast majority of predictions are made under conditions of severe time constraints (a few hours of clinician time per subject), unavailability of important informants, and incomplete archival records. Clinicians asked or required to make predictions rarely have investigative resources that extend into the health care system, criminal justice system, and community. The "subject," that is, the individual about whom one might make a prediction (including patients, suspects, defendants, probationers, and parolees), is never a sufficient source of information for a judgment that he or she will not engage in future crime; the subject may be a sufficient source of information for a positive prediction. If, as is usually the case, the subject is brought to the clinician's attention by someone else, it is essential that this other person's information be sought. Too often a judge, lawyer, or law enforcement officer refers or brings a subject for evaluation without providing the information that has already been gathered, on the assumption that the clinician will somehow discern it. A clinician should never offer a prediction of future criminality without knowing in detail the reason the prediction is sought and should never offer a negative prediction without obtaining all information about the index offense and the official record of the subject's criminal history (Kozol, Boucher, & Garofalo, 1972).

A comprehensive assessment of future criminality could include multiple interviews with the subject, interviews with many of the subject's social contacts (e.g., parents, spouse, siblings, children, co-workers, supervisors, and friends), living victims of current and past offenses, witnesses to the index offense, and the arresting officers. The staff who have worked with the subject, if in confinement, often are in possession of important information. Criminal, correctional, hospital, medical, military, employment, and school records may each be important. Moreover, social contacts and records from each of the subject's previous habitats may prove relevant, because the population at issue is characterized by high geographic mobility. The criminal history should include not only the arrest record, but also police reports from all investigations, probation and parole officers' reports, and records from jails, prisons, and forensic facilities. Sources of information that are too rarely pursued are visits to crime scenes, inspection of crime scene and victim photographs, and visits to the subject's lodgings and workplace. Psychological testing, electroencephalography, biochemical tests, sodium amytal interviews, hypnosis, polygraphy, and penile plethysmography should be available for use in some cases.

In practice, this complete range of sources of information is almost never consulted. At a minimum it would take several weeks of effort to complete the evaluation of a single case if each of these sources were to be pursued. Yet there are other kinds of clinical situations in which the investment of resources is every bit that great. Many medical and surgical patients are evaluated at a cost in excess of what this full-scale evaluation would cost. The fact that "dangerousness" assessments, even in academic centers, are not conducted with this degree of thoroughness is an important indication of the current level of investment of societal resources in making clinical predictions of violence.[8] The fact that comprehensive evaluations are rarely undertaken is important to bear in mind in evaluating empirical studies of the validity of prediction. The major studies showing poor predictions are frequently interpreted by others, if not by their authors, as demonstrating the inability of clinicians to make predictions. Many of these studies have focused on inmates evaluated at public hospitals for the criminally insane (Steadman & Cocozza, 1974; Thornberry & Jacoby, 1979) and special institutions for personality-disordered offenders (Kozol et al., 1972; Steadman, 1977).[9] Judging our clinical predictive capacities on the basis of outcomes for inmates discharged from institutions for the criminally insane is like evaluating current medical technology on the basis of the infant mortality rate in Third World countries.

The process of evaluation

The clinician seeking a list of signs, symptoms, or other predictors of future violence will find extraordinarily meager guidance from texts on general psychiatry or psychology, forensic psychiatry or psychology, or violence. More has been written about our inability to make such predictions and the reasons such predictions should not be made than has been written about how we can responsibly attempt such predictions. The lack of practical advice reflects at least six forces working against those who would offer such guidance.

The first of these is a reluctance to offer opinions that are not substantiated by empirical research. This force must be weak, for it does not prevent clinicians from making predictions in individual cases. The second is the understandable reluctance of those who mount the witness stand to disseminate opinions that, however carefully thought out, are certain to err by commission and omission, to be subject to change, and to return to haunt their authors through cross-examination at a later date. The third force is a reluctance to fly in the face of the opinion of so many eminent authorities that the task is impossible and should not be undertaken. The fourth is the sense that there is so sizable a body of literature purporting to be devoted to the subject of dangerousness and the prediction of violence that it would not be responsible to offer opinions on matters that have been so widely discussed without consulting the preexisting body of knowledge and opinions.[10] The fifth force is the confusing nature of the existing literature, which shows little consistency in definitions, variables, measurements, or contexts.[11] The sixth and least remedial of the forces preventing formalization of clinical guidelines is the inherent complexity of the task. Each of us who renders clinical opinions about future violence does so through mechanisms that reflect our personal backgrounds, training, social roles, institutional roles, attitudes, values, and beliefs. Leaving aside the question of whether it is proper that our opinions should be influenced by all of these variables, it is clear that the transmission of this complex decision-making process from one person to another is a difficult task.[12]

Initially, the most important objective is to obtain, through whatever sources are available, a detailed description of every crime that can be attributed to the subject. Knowing the criminal code labels of the subject's previous convictions is not sufficient. First, many subjects have committed crimes for which they were not arrested. Second, the category of crime for which a subject was convicted cannot be assumed to be an accurate representation of the crime that was actually committed. In a great many cases plea bargaining, evidentiary shortcomings, and prosecutorial discretion will have reduced several applicable charges to a smaller number of less serious charges. Third, certain important elements of an offense cannot be discerned simply from the legal name of the offense. A conviction for assault and battery can mean anything from involvement in a barroom brawl to sadistic torture of a victim. Likewise, an armed robbery conviction can mean anything from threatening a convenience store clerk with a rubber knife to abducting a taxi driver at gunpoint, leaving him tied up in a field, and shooting him.

It is an extremely common error to accept the subject's description of the offense at face value. Despite an apparent willingness to talk about the offense, subjects whom the author has examined have included one who neglected to mention the slashing of clothing in the home of a woman he burglarized, another who failed to report having recorded a torture victim's screams, and a third who did not reveal a nightly ritual of stalking the neighborhood in battle fatigues armed with several weapons. To make matters worse, details such as these are precisely those that everyone else "forgets" to mention, sometimes because they are not recognized as being important, sometimes in order to increase their dramatic value at the trial, and sometimes because they have been repressed or are considered too unseemly to mention. Yet this is the kind of information that should carry the greatest weight in a prediction of criminal behavior.

Identifying and weighting the predictor variables

The clinician attempting to assess an individual's likelihood of committing an intolerable crime (the criterion variable) ideally would be able to specify the predictor variables relied upon and to estimate a quantitative probability but would search in vain for guidance on these matters in the statutes assuming this ability, the court orders demanding this activity, or the judicial decisions proclaiming that such things are possible. According to Roth (1981), skilled practitioners refine their actuarial predictions (assumptions about base rates) by incorporating correction factors based on their previous observations of certain features in similar cases that enable them to assign the individual in question to a known subclass.[13] Although "the task of apportioning the appropriate weight to the different groups of features that have some predictive value" is generally one for the clinician's brain, Roth (1981) expresses hope that "such prediction methods can become a less private and more publicly shared process that is subject to independent evaluation" (p. 105).

In the following pages, I set forth one set of predictive hypotheses. These personal hypotheses should not be adopted as guidelines for clinical work. Their sources (in order of decreasing influence) are *unsystematic* observation, familiarity with the clinical and research literature, experience in several empirical studies of offenders, and familiarity with national crime statistics. The observations have been made chiefly in standard clinical settings (emergency rooms, clinics, and hospitals) and specialized clinical settings (forensic clinics, security hospitals, and prisons) in which individuals whose past offenses are partially known, and whose subsequent offenses occasionally become known, are examined. Another source of observations of a different nature strongly colors these hypotheses, and that is the privilege afforded me of studying crimes with members of the FBI Academy Behavioral Science Unit, where information about a crime is used to predict the characteristics of the offender and where follow-up information to confirm or (less often) disconfirm the prediction is frequently available. In many of these cases the offender remained at large, committing repeated crimes, before the case was referred to the FBI. Familiarity with such cases and with detailed life histories of individual criminals recorded by clinicians in the nineteenth and early twentieth centuries (especially the works of Krafft-Ebing, Jacobus X, Bloch, Wulffen, Stekel, and Karpman) provides outcome information that is unavailable from standard clinical experience. An important shortcoming of such information is that the degree to which a case is extreme and unrepresentative is positively correlated with its probability of referral, publication, and memorability. Thus, I have had to struggle against the tendency to overestimate the weight of predictor variables in formulating these hypotheses.

Although it might be hoped that familiarity with national crime statistics would help one attend to base rates and that familiarity with and experience in empirical research might protect one against incorporating illusory correlations into one's beliefs, there is no measure or guarantee of these effects. The evidence reviewed by Monahan (1981) convincingly demonstrates that the tendencies to ignore base rates and to rely on illusory correlations are widespread psychological processes, and it may be that awareness of these tendencies does little to reduce them.

Hypotheses are, of course, an inadequate substitute for empirical research, but clinicians are compelled by courts and other institutions to play their "hunches" even when no research is available to inform their judgments as to the predictive value of features observed clinically. Moreover, as will be clear from the first group of predictors listed, customary forms of research are not possible for some hypothesized predictors because individuals known to have these features are usually incarcerated for lengthy periods.

In order that the "hunches" presented here be susceptible to empirical disproof (to the extent that the requisite measurements could be made), it is necessary to specify the predictor variables, the criterion variable, and the hypothesized level of association between them. Level of association is conceptualized here as three mutually exclusive ranges that define first-, second-, and third-rank predictors. These ranges are hypothesized probabilities that an individual will engage in any intolerable crime at some time in the future if not incarcerated. First-rank predictors are those for which the probability is estimated to be $>.50$ (50%); for second-rank predictors, $.10 \leq p \leq .50$ (10–50%); and for third-rank predictors, the probability is estimated to be greater than two times the base rate of the general population (which is of the order of .00002), but less than .10 (0.004–10%).

First-rank predictor variables are those believed to be so highly and specifically associated with the criterion variable (i.e., commission of any intolerable crime) that the presence of a single predictor is sufficient for a positive prediction. Each of the predictors specified has a low prevalence, but any one of them is hypothesized to define a population with a probability of future intolerable crime of greater than 50%. If the hypothesized probabilities within these populations, so defined, are correct, then the most accurate prediction would be that all individuals with any first-rank predictor are positive.

The following are examples of hypothesized first-rank predictors:

1. One murder with mutilation of the corpse
2. One murder with vampirism
3. One murder with cannibalism
4. One murder with antemortem sexual sadism
5. One contract murder
6. One sniper murder of a stranger
7. One abduction with torture of the victim
8. Three forcible rapes of strangers
9. One arson episode with sexual arousal
10. Two arson episodes for profit
11. One kidnapping for ransom
12. One bombing of an occupied building
13. Two bombings of motor vehicles
14. One forcible rape with torture of the victim
15. Two episodes in which a child under 12 was forcibly raped or tortured
16. One instance of insertion of the penis in a body orifice of an infant
17. Three batteries of an individual child under 12
18. Three batteries of a spouse within 1 year
19. Three or more felonious assaultive acts within 1 year with escalating degrees of violence
20. Two unprovoked attacks on strangers with a lethal weapon
21. Five violent offenses of any kind
22. Threats to kill another named person uttered three or more times, at least two of which included no display of anger, and extending over a period of at least 3 months
23. Preoccupation with a casual acquaintance or stranger lasting more than 3 months with at least one attempt at direct communication with the other person and at least one potentially injurious action directed at the other person, a surrogate for the other person, someone believed to be associated with the other person, or an effigy or symbol of the other person
24. A plan to commit an intolerable crime that the subject says he or she fully intends to carry out and a history of any violent felony
25. Delusional beliefs not acknowledged as delusional by the subject that, if true, would justify an intolerable crime and a history of any violent felony and a history of stopping medication against medical advice

Second-rank predictors are those believed to define populations with a probability of committing intolerable crime of between 10 and 50%. If this is correct, the individual faced with a decision about what to do with a person with one such feature faces a dilemma. It would be most accurate to predict all such persons to be negatives, but because the criterion variable is commission of an intolerable crime, it may be preferable to risk having 1 to 10 false positives for each true positive prediction by predicting all positive. If all were predicted negative, 10 to 50% would be false negatives. Whether this or any other specifiable probability is great enough to justify preventive intervention is a social policy question to be left to judges and legislators (Monahan & Wexler, 1978). The following are examples of hypothesized second-rank predictors:

1. One firearm offense within the preceding year
2. One forcible rape within the preceding year
3. One burglary with destruction of female clothing or bedding, killing of a pet, theft of fetish items, or writing on a wall or mirror
4. Sadistic sexual fantasies and a history of any violent felony
5. One attempted or completed arson
6. One attempted or completed abduction
7. Any offense in which the victim was bound
8. The purchase of a weapon with a threat or plan to harm someone
9. One offense the initial intent of which was to acquire material goods but which came to involve unnecessary violence when something did not go according to plan
10. One episode of brutality toward an unresisting victim during the commission of another offense
11. Two batteries against anyone in the home within the past year
12. Two batteries within a residential institution within the past year
13. Use of a lethal weapon in the intentional destruction of an effigy or symbol of a family member or lover or such person's property within the past year
14. Morbid jealousy with a history of any violent offense
15. Alcoholism and any violent offense within the past year
16. Alcoholism and a habit of carrying a lethal weapon
17. One episode of unlawfully cutting another person with a knife
18. One episode of unlawfully drugging or poisoning another person
19. Keeping a diary describing past crimes
20. Tape recording the victim's utterances in a previous offense
21. A diagnosis of antisocial personality disorder with at least one arrest for a violent offense
22. A diagnosis of paranoid schizophrenia with a history of at least two violent acts while psychotic and at least two episodes of stopping neuroleptic medication against medical advice
23. A history of being abused during childhood coupled with an arrest for any violent offense
24. Use of a lethal weapon at any time in the interest of preserving an ongoing, profitable, unlawful enterprise (e.g., pimping, prostitution, or drug dealing)
25. Three violent offenses of any kind

Third-rank predictors complicate the picture immeasurably. These are predictor variables believed to define populations with a probability of committing an intolerable crime that is at least twofold greater than that of the general population, but still less than 10%. Thus, the probabilities for these populations might be as low as .004% or as high as 10%. Although a few of these items (e.g., 9, 10, and 14) are unlawful under some circumstances, the others would certainly not be considered a sufficient basis for confinement of an individual without mental disorder (at least in North America). Yet the first several of these have been empirically established as better actuarial predictors of future violence than the diagnosis of any psychotic mental disorder. Mental illness may be as unreasonable a predicate condition for preventive detention as any of these hypothesized third-rank predictors:

1. Has a juvenile record
2. Has a felony record
3. Is male
4. Age is 16 to 24
5. Is black
6. Is poor
7. Father is absent from family of origin
8. Has a tattoo
9. Possesses a cheap handgun
10. Has a gun collection
11. Has a preference for bondage and domination pornography
12. Reads detective magazines
13. Reads mercenary and terrorist magazines
14. Owns child pornography
15. Collects Nazi memorabilia
16. Has sought out work with the wounded in an accident department or ambulance service
17. Has sought out work with the dead in a morgue or funeral home
18. Has sought out flesh-incising work in a butcher shop, slaughter house, or operating theater
19. Has worked as a private security guard or auxiliary police officer
20. Has worked as a volunteer fireman
21. Has been a paid employee in a police, fire, or correctional department in association with any personality disorder or sexual deviation
22. Has been or is associated with an extremist political organization
23. Is preoccupied with inner fantasies to the detriment of social functioning
24. Has a first-degree relative with a criminal record
25. Has a history of threatening and filing lawsuits that have never succeeded

Each of the predictor variables mentioned so far is such that it could be reliably documented, although some, such as delusions or fantasies of a specific nature, cannot always be validly detected. To these one might add a sizable number of temperamental and personality traits that challenge not only our powers of valid detection, but also our capacity to define reliably without cumbersome procedures. The following are examples of such predictors:

1. Incapacity to feel sympathy
2. Inability to learn from experience
3. Impulsivity
4. Narcissistic traits
5. Paranoid traits
6. Borderline traits
7. Inner rage
8. Overcontrolled aggression
9. External locus of control
10. Hypertrophied sense of injustice

Scott (1977) emphasizes the first two of these (incapacity to feel sympathy and to learn from experience), but they, like the others among these psychological constructs, ought to be regarded as "soft signs." Soft signs are observations on which clinicians may reasonably rely but that must be documented by psychological testing or a description of what one means by them along with examples of the observed behavior that leads one to conclude that they are present. If these soft signs are predictive at all, they are surely not first- or second-rank predictors.

Assuming for argument's sake that the hypothetical predictors and weights set forth here are accurate, the questions remain as to which of these public policy should allow to be used for making predictions and, of these, how they are to be combined to render predictions. Should sex, race, and poverty be permissible bases for such predictions? Should those who exercise the right to collect guns, to read particular types of magazines, or to associate with extremist political groups be "penalized" for so doing? Should surgeons, nurses, orderlies, butchers, security guards, and volunteer firemen be "penalized" on the basis of their callings?

Given a list of acceptable predictors, each of which could be shown to have a zero-order relationship to intolerable crime, what would we accept as adequate evidence of their impact in a multivariate analysis? Ideally, I suppose we should look for total explained variance for a given set of predictors with respect to a single criterion offense, but there is no end to the permutations that could be tried in searching for the best equations.

Conclusions

This exercise in articulating personal "hunches" was undertaken with the expectation that an effort to make public such beliefs might result in the formulation of testable hypotheses. To some extent this has been accomplished, although, as noted, not all can be tested in the conventional manner. Beyond this, however, it should be disclosed that in the process of committing these ideas to paper (while self-consciously attempting to guard against the common errors of clinical prediction) I have found that many previously held beliefs about the predictive significance of specific variables have melted away under the imagined glare of public scrutiny. One observation that can be made on the basis of this exercise is that those who are required to render opinions about "dangerousness" might profit from similar efforts to articulate their assumptions and underlying beliefs.

It seems to me that first-rank predictors are obvious enough that most decision makers would rely on them regardless of clinical opinion or empirical evidence. Among the second-rank predictors, however, some are given less weight than I believe would be warranted if their importance were more widely recognized.

Whether a predictor should be a sufficient basis for confinement is not, of course, for clinicians to say, but must be an individualized judgment that takes account of many other factors, including the length of confinement. These judgments should be most difficult when a second-rank predictor is the strongest predictive evidence available. The task for clinicians and researchers is to identify, verify, and articulate to policy makers the nature and probabilistic importance of predictors. Second-rank predictors have the highest priority for this work.

The possible uses of first-, second-, and third-rank predictors in civil commitment of the mentally ill deserve comment. In civil commitment proceedings concerning individuals who have a first-rank predictor, the fact finder will generally need no convincing about the individual's potential for harming others (assuming that testimony about the index offense or behavior is admissible). The challenge to the party seeking commitment under current statutes should be that of attributing this potential to mental disease or defect. The reason that this should be challenging is that the danger in most cases has little or nothing to do with mental disease or defect, but rather reflects some combination of inadequate socialization, environmental impoverishment, and personality traits (including sexual deviation).[14]

In civil commitment proceedings concerning individuals who have only a second-rank predictor, the party seeking commitment has an additional challenge, namely, that of convincing the fact finder that a probability of 10 to 50% is sufficient to justify commitment. In this respect, current statutory language varies widely. Decision makers would do well to take note that predictions at a higher level of probability can be made only in the most obvious cases.

It should also be noted that nearly all of the predictors mentioned here have to do with phenomena that are not discussed in the traditional curricula for medicine, psychiatry, or psychology. Although they are for the most part criminological, they have to do with individual criminality, a subject given little attention in the criminology courses and degree programs in sociology departments and schools of public administration. Karpman's (1940) effort to focus interest on individual criminality and to define and promote a discipline of criminal psychopathology never took root, although clinicians and researchers from various disciplines have continued to make important contributions.

Whatever limited abilities clinicians have in the prediction of crime reflects their knowledge of criminals, criminality, crime, and criminology more than their credentialed knowledge of psychiatry or psychology. Psychiatrists and psychologists who have no knowledge of crime have no more business predicting crime than other citizens. Yet members of other disciplines that do not subject their members to professional socialization practices designed to foster responsibility for one's judgments should not be empowered to deprive people of their liberty through such judgments, whatever their knowledge of crime may be. For the most part, those who have the power lack the relevant knowledge, whereas those with the relevant knowledge lack power.

Perhaps one day the clinical prediction of intolerable crime will be a task for the as yet unrecognized specialty of clinical criminology.[15] In the meantime, a body of variously informed clinicians, most of whom have only minimal knowledge of crime, will remain empowered and expected by the courts and the public to make professional judgments about matters beyond their competence.[16] Some, of course, seek to acquire expertise about "dangerousness" (although rarely about crime). Many others, unfortunately, are content to accept the false assumption by the courts and public that they are, indeed, experts in the prediction of criminal conduct. The confidence man's work is not legitimized by the abundance of eager victims. To predict criminal behavior without knowledge of crime is a psycholegal confidence game.

Notes

1 Most of these are "intolerable crimes" because they are perceived to be predictable.
2 Prediction of crime is merely one of the tasks through which clinicians can and should promote injury control. The forensic pathologist whose autopsy suggests a source of carbon monoxide poisoning in an apartment building, the pediatrician who instructs parents on electrical socket guards, and the public health officer who works to modify highway hazards are all performing comparable functions. For a discussion directed to surgeons, see Baker and Dietz (1979).

  The paternalistic and self-protective purposes of prediction are also interesting and important, but they depend on the particulars of the relationships between the predictor, the subject, and the institutions (such as hospitals, prisons, and courts) in which predictions are made. These relationships are founded on tradition (e.g., the physician–patient relationship), law (e.g., psychotherapist–client privilege), and administrative circumstances (e.g., the party by whom the predictor is retained). Each of these foundations is a source of bias to be guarded against in rendering predictions for injury control purposes, as well as a major consideration when paternalistic and self-protective purposes are simultaneously entertained.
3 This discussion is arbitrarily limited to the prediction of crimes, thereby excluding self-destructive behaviors.
4 Statutory and case law governing involuntary commitment promulgate various concepts of danger or harm to others. Although these are of immense practical significance, in the broader view they are folkways and should be regarded as neither immutable nor the necessary starting point of a fresh inquiry. Moreover, if we allow ourselves to be diverted to a consideration of prediction for the purpose of civil commitment, we shall follow the well-trodden path by which many others have lost sight of the fact that such predictive abilities as we have are not necessarily those expected by law. Those readers who seek guidance as to how to predict whether an individual will commit *any* act that might result in bodily harm to another will be disappointed in what follows. Perhaps a few unusually talented and intuitive clinicians make such predictions well, but it is doubtful that the process by which they do so could ever be systematized.

  My justification for sidestepping the types of predictions customarily demanded of us is threefold. First, I do not believe that dangerousness should be necessary for civil commitment of the mentally ill, although I think it should be among the available bases for commitment. Second, to the extent that our concern is with crime prevention, I regard civil commitment of the mentally ill as a low-priority strategy. Third, like Kittrie (1979), I am puzzled that dangerousness should be regarded as justifying preventive detention only among the mentally ill. I suppose this to be a remnant of the paternalism that is being purged from so much of mental health law and an indication that the formulators of such policy assume the mentally ill as a class to be unsusceptible to the deterrence assumed for criminal sanctions. These assumptions need reevaluation. Not all mental disorders impair susceptibility to deterrence, and those that do so have effects that vary in nature and degree. Moreover, mental disorder is by no means the only recognizable factor that can impair susceptibility to deterrence.

5 Aware of the circularity of this last group, I considered entitling this chapter "The Prediction of Predictable Crimes."

6 Such crimes are increasingly the basis of tort actions against clinicians and hospital authorities and against parole boards and other correctional authorities. As already noted, however, the self-protective function of prediction is not the focus of this chapter.

7 This does not mean that the average citizen, given a choice between having these crimes and not having them, would choose to have them. It means that the collective citizenry, given the choice between the freedoms that promote these crimes and the restrictions that would reduce them, has thus far opted to retain the freedoms with their attendant costs.

8 Because the value of full-scale evaluations is currently unknown, the required expenditures would not be justified as a matter of routine. An investment in research that would measure this value would, however, be justified.

9 For readers unfamiliar with such institutions, an illustration might be useful. For a decade it has been known that the better actuarial predictors of postrelease violence include the presence of a juvenile record, the number of previous arrests, the presence of previous convictions for violent crimes, and the severity of the index offense (Steadman & Cocozza, 1973). Despite this knowledge, data on none of these four items are routinely made available to practitioners in Massachusetts performing court-ordered evaluations of "dangerousness" (at a frequency of more than 600 such assessments per year at Bridgewater State Hospital alone). Data on juvenile records and previous convictions are not available because an efficient means of obtaining these from other agencies has never been established. Data on previous arrests are unavailable because there are no adequate arrest records in Massachusetts (although Probation Department records contain good data on court appearances and thus reflect most of the arrests that reach that stage). Data on the severity of the index offense are inadequate because courts often provide only a partial list of offenses charged, sometimes omitting the most serious ones, and because police departments ignore requests for police reports. Nonetheless, clinical opinions on "dangerousness" are ordered and delivered.

Moving accounts of life among the inmates of such institutions are to be found in Rawls (1980), Thomas & Stebel (1980), and the film *Titicut Follies*.

10 Those who find themselves in the business of predicting violence most often conduct it at a considerable distance from that luxurious and civilized institution known as the library, a distance measured not only in miles, but also in time, access, and inclination. It is an unpleasant fact of life that those who choose to work in settings where the prediction of violence is an everyday necessity tend to be of the nonreading persuasion. Those who are of the nonreading persuasion, thankfully, tend also to be of the nonwriting persuasion.

11 The remedy for this confusion is Monahan's monograph, *The Clinical Prediction of Violent Behavior* (1981). Monahan lays out existing knowledge and its deficits so clearly and with such faithful attention to the methodological strengths and weaknesses of empirical studies that his book can serve as the proper starting point for all subsequent considerations of the relevant issues.

12 This task is perhaps analogous to attempting to teach another person to come reliably to the same conclusion as oneself with regard to which and how many of a group of new acquaintances should be regarded as desirable dinner companions.

13 Physicians may be reminded here of the identification of unknown samples in chemistry laboratories. From some of the properties of a substance, its composition can be ascertained, thereby

allowing one to predict its "behavior" under conditions not yet tested. To the inexperienced, these properties are observable but meaningless, but the expert learns to predict "behavior" on the basis of observations of these properties. How could a chemist function if the properties of known substances were so variable that, having identified a sample, he or she could say no more than that there was a 50% probability that it would behave as a corrosive acid and a 50% probability that it would behave as water? And if the same sample could sometimes behave as an acid, sometimes as water, depending on unpredictable and unmeasurable extraneous circumstances, how could the chemist make a pot of coffee?

14 This view is not widely shared.

15 For the moment, the only sensible route to becoming a clinical criminologist is to acquire credentials in one of the empowered, recognized fields, namely, psychiatry or psychology, and to acquire knowledge of crime through other means. These include the formal study of criminology, self-education in criminology, and experience in working with criminals and the criminal justice system.

Ideally, the clinical criminologist will draw on all of these sources of knowledge. Unfortunately, we provide little incentive to seek such knowledge. Those who acquire it do so at their own expense yet find that there are no attractive career paths available that would have been otherwise unavailable. No salary rewards are forthcoming as a result of the additional knowledge and experience. Occasionally, such a clinician's testimony will carry greater weight in court, but for the most part any "expert" will do. And what of the criminologist who is motivated to seek clinical credentials? After a long and expensive period of training, he or she would find a new range of career opportunities available. How many would then choose to work with criminal populations?

16 Many clinicians are appropriately uncomfortable with these powers and expectations. Such individuals should request consultation whenever in doubt. It will be interesting to see whether nonspecialists will be held to a lesser standard of care in malpractice cases, now that board certification is available in forensic psychiatry and forensic psychology.

References

Baker, S. P., & Dietz, P. E. The epidemiology and prevention of injuries. In G. D. Zuidema, R. B. Rutherford, & W. F. Ballinger II (Eds.), *The management of trauma* (3rd ed.). Philadelphia: Saunders, 1979.

Karpman, B. The principles and aims of criminal psychopathology. *Criminal Psychopathology*, 1940, *1*, 187–218.

Kittrie, N. N. The prediction of dangerousness: The experts, the courts, and the criminal justice system. In N. J. Beran & B. G. Toomey (Eds.), *Mentally ill offenders and the criminal justice system: Issues in forensic services.* New York: Praeger, 1979.

Kozol, H. L., Boucher, R. J., & Garofalo, R. F. The diagnosis and treatment of dangerousness. *Crime and Delinquency*, 1972, *18*, 371–92.

Monahan, J. *The clinical prediction of violent behavior* (DHHS Publication No. [ADM] 81–921). Washington, D.C.: U.S. Government Printing Office, 1981.

Monahan, J., & Wexler, D. B. A definite maybe: Proofs and probability in civil commitment. *Law and Human Behavior*, 1978, *2*, 37–42.

Rawls, W., Jr. *Cold storage.* New York: Simon & Schuster, 1980.

Roth, M. Modern psychiatry and neurology and the problem of responsibility. In S. J. Hucker, C. D. Webster, & M. H. Ben-Aron (Eds.), *Mental disorder and criminal responsibility.* Toronto: Butterworths, 1981.

Scott, P. D. Assessing dangerousness in criminals. *British Journal of Psychiatry*, 1977, *131*, 127–42.

Steadman, H. J. A new look at recidivism among Patuxent inmates. *Bulletin of the American Academy of Psychiatry and the Law*, 1977, *5*, 200–9.

Steadman, H. J., & Cocozza, J. J. *Careers of the criminally insane*. Lexington, Mass.: Heath, 1974.

Steadman, H. J., & Cocozza, J. J. The criminally insane patient: Who gets out? *Social Psychiatry*, 1973, *8*, 230–8.

Thomas, B. & Stebel, S. L. *The shoe leather treatment*. Los Angeles: Tarcher, 1980.

Thornberry, T. P., & Jacoby, J. E. *The criminally insane: A community follow-up of mentally ill offenders*. Chicago: University of Chicago Press, 1979.

7 A systems approach to the prediction of wife assault: relevance to criminal justice system policy

Donald G. Dutton

Writers seem as much to agree on the historicity of wife assault and uxoricide as they seem to disagree on their causes. Taylor (1954), de Reincourt (1974), Davidson (1977), and Metzger (1980) all note that evidence for both killing and assault of wives[1] appears continuously from earliest recorded history. Medieval tracts such as Gratian's theological manual *The Decretum* (c. 114) declared women to be inferior to men and made explicit the expectation that a husband's duty was to punish (*castigare*) his wife "for correction." The roots of such misogyny were carried to the extreme in the *Malleus Maleficarum* of Heinrich Kramer and Jacob Sprenger, written in 1486, which parlayed presumed female susceptibility to external forces (i.e., devils) and the need for male-applied "correction" into the rationale for medieval witchhunts. Women who incurred male wrath for any of a variety of reasons (including male impotence) were at peril of being burned at the stake. At the same time, women who lived up to the male ideal of femininity were venerated by *l'amour courtoise* (Hunt, 1959) and inundated with a blend of adoration and unconsummated desire. Not until William Heale's "An Apology for Women" (1609) and John Stuart Mill's *The Subjection of Women* (1869) does one see public written protests by men of the physical and political subjugation of women. By the 1890s wife assault was de jure illegal under British common law and in some U.S. states. To this day, it is de facto legal to the extent that it is largely ignored as a serious crime by the criminal justice system.

The widespread incidence of violent crimes against women has been reported in a variety of sources and should no longer require documentation. Straus, Gelles, and Steinmetz (1977) uncovered "violent episodes" in 28% of a sample of 2,143 self-reported "happily married couples."[2] Virtually all clinical reports would indicate that both men (in order to minimize responsibility or because of poor memory; see Dutton, 1982; Szinovacz, 1983) and women (Dutton & Painter, 1981) tend to underreport violence in intimate relationships. A survey of women in Kentucky revealed that only 8.6% of wife assaults were reported to the police (Schulman, 1980).

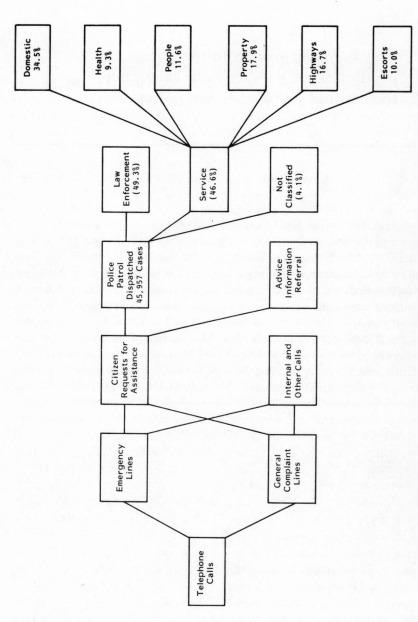

Figure 7.1. Telephone requests for police assistance and breakdown of dispatches into "service" and "law enforcement." Adapted from Levens and Dutton (1980, p. 21) and reproduced by kind permission of the Solicitor General, Canada.

Table 7.1. *Distribution of "service" dispatches by subgroup, time taken, and number of calls, January to June 1975*

Type of service call	Total calls		Total time (min)		Average time per case (min)
	No.	%	No.	%	
Domestic	7,396	34.5	234,811	24.3	31.8
Health	1,994	9.3	114,752	11.9	57.6
People	2,491	11.6	69,739	7.2	28.0
Property	3,838	17.9	183,211	19.0	47.9
Highways	3,573	16.7	291,790	30.2	81.7
Escorts	2,137	10.0	71,725	7.4	33.6
Total services	21,419	100.0	966,028	100.0	45.1

Source: Levens and Dutton (1980, p. 22).

Despite this reluctance to involve the police, the largest category of calls for police service are "domestic dispute calls" (Levens & Dutton, 1977). This is apparent in Figure 7.1 and Table 7.1. With the exception of some innovative programs (Dutton, 1982), the response of the criminal justice system to wife assault has been weak. Only about one-half of the calls for service are answered (Levens & Dutton, 1980) and police reports, which are usually required by a justice of the peace before laying on information (laying a charge), are written by police in only a minority (18%) of cases (Levens & Dutton, 1980). Hence, if a woman has called the police for assistance, she has only 1 chance out of 10 that they will attend and write the requisite report allowing a justice of the peace to lay on information.

My research on the response of the criminal justice system to wife assault and the attitudinal constraints that operate against a more active policy of prosecuting wife assaulters has been described in detail elsewhere (Dutton, 1977, 1981, 1982; Levens & Dutton, 1980). By combining Schulman's (1980) victim survey with Parnas's (1973) and Leven and Dutton's (1980) studies of attrition rates for criminal justice system prosecution of wife assault, I estimated that, for every 10,000 wife assaults, only 2 result in convictions (Table 7.2). Of course, these studies were done in three different jurisdictions, selected on the basis of availability to the researcher. Hence, we have only the reports of practitioners to suggest their representativeness (U.S. Commission on Civil Rights, 1978). Police reluctance to adopt a more aggressive policy of prosecution against wife assaulters stems from the belief that the woman will drop the charges or that the crown prosecutor will not readily proceed except in the most extreme cases. Of course, the latter "cause" is a classic example of "blaming the victim" (Ryan, 1971), which establishes a self-fulfilling prophecy operating against state intervention on be-

Table 7.2. *Attrition rates in the criminal justice system for wife assault cases*

Outcome	Reference
10,000 assaults	Schulman (1980) (revealed by victim survey)
860 reported to police	Schulman (1980)
420 police responses	Levens and Dutton (1980)
49 warrants for arrest	Parnas (1973)
3 cases proceeded with	Parnas (1973)
2 convictions	Parnas (1973)

half of assaulted women (see Dutton, 1982). The reluctance of the police to be more involved in wife assault cases reflects the general societal attitude that violence between husband and wife is a "private affair" (Shotland & Straw, 1976; Stark & McEvoy, 1970), is not serious, and will resolve itself with the partners "making up." Shotland and Straw (1976), for example, found that, when onlookers believed a male–female conflict to be betweeen a married couple, they believed the woman to be in less danger (although the conflict was becoming physical), to be less likely to want their help, and to be less likely to aid them against the man if they did help, than in an identical conflict between apparent strangers. Only 19% attempted to intervene in any way, compared with 69% who believed that the conflict was between strangers.

The police view their mandate as being to quiet the conflict for the evening, with little thought of the probability of recidivism or the possibility of escalating severity in future assaults. Yet a study funded by the Police Foundation in Washington, D.C. (Wilt & Breedlove, 1977) revealed that, in serious cases of felonious assault (comparable to assault causing bodily harm in Canada) or murder, police had been called to the address where the offense occurred at least once before in 90% of the offenses or five or more times before in 50% of the offenses. These data may suggest a pattern of repeated assault, escalating in severity, and argue against the use of mere short-term measures in family conflict resolution. They raise the question of whether an assault between intimates who remain in contact is likely to be repeated. Given that the conflict underlying the assault has not been resolved, that the assault may have served a variety of rewarding functions for the assaultive party (Dutton, Fehr, & McEwan, 1982; Novaco, 1976), and that the assaulter has not been punished by arrest and conviction, this repetition is likely in theory. With our present lack of knowledge about baseline rates for wife assault, however, we do not know the percentage of wife assaults that are not repeated and the percentage of those that escalate to the point of coming to the attention of the criminal justice system. We do know that, if an assault was reported to the police and did not proceed to court, the chances of a repeated assault involving the same parties within a very short time is 67%. If the case did proceed to court, the recidivism rate drops to 30% irrespective of the disposition (Jaffe, 1982).

The causes of wife assault

Throughout the 1970s, when the seminal studies on wife assault were done (cf. Dobash & Dobash, 1979; Elbow, 1977; Gelles, 1974; Rounsaville, 1978; Steinmetz & Straus, 1974; Straus, 1973, 1976, 1977a,b; Symonds, 1978; Whitehurst, 1974), two prevalent theories of the etiology of wife assault were that (a) wife assault was normative behavior in a sexist society, that in Straus's words "a marriage licence is a hitting licence" (Straus, 1977a,b); (b) wife assault was a sign of psychiatric disturbance, "neurotic character development" (Symonds, 1978, p. 219), or "conjugal paranoia" (*Diagnostic and Statistical Manual of the Mental Disorders,* 1980, p. 195). The evidence would seem to suggest that both the sociological and psychiatric explanations are incomplete.

Data relevant to the normative nature of wife assault come from a survey conducted by Stark and McEvoy (1970) for the U.S. National Commission on the Causes and Prevention of Violence, which revealed that one in four men and one in six women approved of a husband slapping a wife under "appropriate circumstances." Straus (1976) has interpreted these results as representative of normative acceptance of violence toward women. Some caveats are in order, however. First, slapping is not the same as beating or assault. Presumably, far fewer people would approve as the violent act became more extreme. Second, even at the level of slapping, only 25% of men approve. Despite the widespread incidence of wife assault, it appears that a sizable minority rather than a majority of North American men are assaultive with their wives. The survey of 2,143 U.S. couples by Straus, Gelles, and Steinmetz (1980) suggested that 12.6% had "ever" engaged in an act of severe violence. The "normative" explanation fails to differentiate the assaultive from the nonassaultive man.

Psychiatric explanations of wife assault, however, have to account for evidence which suggests that many assaultive men do not have diagnosable disorders apart from their violence. Rounsaville (1978) and Ganley and Harris (1978) describe assaultive men as impulsive, likely to abuse alcohol, and having problems with dependency–intimacy issues. Rosenbaum and O'Leary (1981) describe assaultive men as less assertive with their wives than were nonassaultive husbands in therapy and as more likely to have witnessed parental spouse abuse. Unfortunately, these studies tend to suffer from two methodological problems: (a) Baseline comparison data from nonassaultive controls have not been frequently available, and (b) assessments of husbands' experiences have often been based on wives' reports; hence, selective factors for differential reporting have been a problem (see Szinovacz, 1983).

A nested ecological theory

Belsky (1980) developed a four-level interactionist theory to account for child maltreatment, which I have adopted to guide my present research on wife assault. A nested ecological theory views wife assault as determined by multiple forces in the individual (ontogenetic level), the current family dynamic (microsystem level), and the relationship of the family unit to the broader culture (macrosystem level). Factors from each of these levels are said to be "nested" within the next broader level in that they are viewed as operating within limits set by the next broader level. I have described these levels extensively elsewhere (Dutton, 1984) and shall focus here on the relevance of specific cross-level interactions to the prediction of wife assault and our current research.

Beginning with the most specific level, that of the individual characteristics of the assaultive man, we are concentrating on the conjunction of two specific traits: (a) the need for social power or control vis à vis the wife and (b) anxiety about changes in intimacy or social–emotional distance in the primary relationship. These have been chosen because of their relevance to both the clinical and empirical data on wife assaulters and relationship changes during time of the assault (see Dutton & Painter, 1981; Ganley & Harris, 1978; Rounsaville, 1978) and their relevance to the social psychological literature, which, for me, provides the clearest articulation of the interaction between individual motives and relationship variables.

Following the work of McClelland (1975) and Winter (1973), we are treating power as a motive in husband–wife relationships. On the basis of clinical reports from batterers and data suggesting that dependency issues are paramount in battering relationships (Dutton & Painter, 1980; Gelles, 1975; Symonds, 1978), we are treating intimacy as the major content issue on which power needs are projected. I envison a "comfort zone" for intimacy not unlike the comfort zones described by the research on personal space (Patterson, 1976; Sommer, 1969). "Invasions" consisting of uncomfortable demands for too little emotional distance generate arousal that can be labeled anxiety (an "engulfment panic") in this schema. Demands for too great an emotional distance generate arousal that can also be labeled anxiety (in this case an "abandonment panic"). Alternatively, such arousal can be labeled anger, an emotion that is more consonant with male sex role expectations. In this schema, anger and violence provide a means for the man to (a) regain control of the power relationship by physical means (future threats and intimidation can be based on one physical incident);

(b) ward off expression of anxiety, which may be incompatible with his sex-role-based self-image, by acting violently and hence generating a feeling of anger that covers up the anxiety; and (c) feel expressive, agentic (i.e., acting successfully in the environment), and powerful (see Novaco, 1976). Hence, "histrionic" anger may provide a behavioral means of overriding feelings of anxiety that are incompatible with a traditional male self-concept. Conceptually, from the husband's point of view the notion of a "safe emotional distance" works like a rubber band and coil spring between him and his wife. As she moves too close the spring pushes her back; as she moves too far away the band pulls her closer (see also Dutton & Painter, 1984). We would expect safe emotional distances to vary from one man to the next, depending on experiences in the family of origin, probably with his mother, and to be affected by aversive life events in the contemporary environment that may shrink the range of the safe emotional distance zone, making both engulfment and abandonment panics more likely. Generally, men will attempt to reestablish the intimacy equilibrium by verbal means, but if communication skills in terms of either verbal ability (Rounsaville, 1978) or assertiveness (Rosenbaum & O'Leary, 1981) are lacking, the man may perceive himself to be losing control of the degree of intimacy and may resort to violence as an ultimate means of control. I think the importance of intimacy issues partially accounts for the high incidence of assault beginning during times of rapid change in social–emotional distance. Both Gelles (1975) and Dutton & Painter (1981) found that 33 to 40% of assaults began during the first pregnancy or during the honeymoon period.

Currently, with Jim Browning, I am examining these hypotheses by showing 8-min videotape scenarios of male–female conflicts to (a) wife assaulters court-directed for therapy, (b) nonassaultive men in therapy, and (c) nonassaultive men not in therapy. The scenarios depict engulfment, abandonment, and neutral scenes from the male point of view in which either the man or the woman is verbally dominating the conflict. Pretesting indicates that control-group men view the dominance and intimacy dimensions as we intended. In the abandonment tapes, for example, the woman announces her intention of visiting another city for the weekend with woman friends. In the ensuing conflict she announces her further plan to join a women's consciousness-raising group. In the male-dominant version of this issue, the man talks her out of both plans. In the female-dominant version, the man attempts to talk the woman out of her plans but fails. The engulfment tapes depict a situation in which a woman complains to her husband about the lack of communication in their marriage and the lack of attention she gets from her spouse. Again, both male- and female-dominant versions exist. Finally, a "neutral" (with respect to intimacy) conflict depicts a couple arguing over the location of their holidays (to be spent together). Subjects are shown either male- or female-dominant tapes (counterbalanced for order of presentation). The strongest self-reports of anger among physically assaultive men occurred in the abandonment conditions.

One long-term objective, apart from our present interest in the causation of wife assault, is to develop some videotapes as standardized tests with broader utility in the assessment of violence potential and of sexual violence potential in particular. We are currently looking for differences between assaultive and non-assaultive men in terms of (a) the psychophysiological reaction to the scenarios, (b) the self-reported label put on the arousal, (c) other differences in the description of the conflict, and (d) some behavioral self-reported data. We are also examining the impact of these scenarios as both anger instigators and potentiators of the response to pornography in an effort to examine possible connections between wife assault and sexual violence.

This research does not assume power needs and intimacy issues to be operating in a vacuum. We have also begun to test power motivation in general (Winter's 1973 measure of n power), adherence to sex role stereotypes and adversarial sexual beliefs (Burt, 1980), verbal skills measures (Curley & O'Leary, 1980; Rathus, 1973), exposure to violent childhood models (Straus Conflict Tactics Scale), and measures of current support networks, marital satisfaction, and general use of violence. According to a nested ecological model, wife assault can be a consequence of the interaction of several factors. The likelihood of wife assault will be high in situations involving a man who (a) has a strong need to control a woman, (b) has exaggerated anxieties about changes in intimacy, (c) has had violent role models, (d) does not have well-developed alternative control skills (the first four situations are ontogenetic), (e) is currently experiencing stress from work demands or unemployment (exosystem stressors) or relationship stress (microsystem stressor), and (f) exists in a culture where "maleness" is in part defined by aggressiveness (macrosystem).

Therapy with wife assaulters

Our treatment program operates with men directed by a judge's probation order from family court connections stemming from wife assault. The program involves group therapy designed to (a) overcome resistance to and denial of responsibility for the violence together with tendencies to minimize the violence, (b) improve the ability to detect and label one's own emotions, (c) improve the ability to communicate feelings, (d) teach alternative behaviors for expressing anger, and (5) teach alternative behaviors for satisfying power motivation.

Confrontation within the group serves the first objective. This might go so far as to involve reading from court records of violence to overcome persistent denial. Obviously, no progress can be made with someone who steadfastly believes he does not have a problem (see also Ganley & Harris, 1978). To improve the ability to detect and express emotion, a variety of techniques are used. Clinicians seem in general agreement that wife assaulters are emotionally "closed," unwilling to express emotion, and often unable to detect what they themselves are feeling. I have personally witnessed men pounding clenched fists into their hands and clenching their jaws as they recounted events leading up to an assault. When asked what they were presently feeling or were feeling at the time, they seemed unable to respond. By having the men keep "anger diaries" in which they note all the events in the course of a week that have angered them, how they interpreted each event (their "internal dialogue"), how angry they became, and how they experienced the anger (physically, emotionally, etc.), some sensitivity to detecting emotions is developed. These techniques stem from a social-learning orientation (Bandura, 1973; Meichenbaum, 1974; Novaco, 1975) that treats violence as a learned response to stress. Where we go beyond a conventional behavior modification approach is in the use of Gestalt and psychodrama to unearth the basis of stressful male–female conflicts. Also, we attempt to bolster assertiveness skills, to initiate holistic life-style management that allows for alternative means of experiencing feelings of power, and to examine sex role beliefs. The immediate goal of this therapy is anger management (cf. Novaco, 1975), superseded by improved communication skills and consciousness raising. Preliminary indications suggest that such therapy can be successful. A systematic evaluation of the treatment outcomes remains to be done.

Prediction of wife assault

As already mentioned, there are theoretical reasons to believe that, once initiated, wife assault will be repeated at intervals. Each assault is self-rewarding: It enables the husband to regain temporary control of a marital struggle, make him feel agentic, expressive, and powerful (cf. Novaco, 1976), and provides pleasurable proprioceptive feedback to an otherwise constricted person (cf. Dutton et al, 1982; Zimbardo, 1969). Furthermore, the inaction of the criminal justice system conveys tacit approval of the actions up to the point at which they become too serious to be ignored. Then, retrospective analyses reveal long histories of assault within the relationship (Martin, 1977), with more than one call to the police for help (Jaffe, 1982; Wilt & Breedlove, 1977). Reconstructed histories of assaultive men reveal high rates of witnessing violence in the family of origin (Rounsaville, 1978). These vicariously learned, long-standing feelings of parental neglect could contribute to the occurrence of assault in the contemporary environment.

Unfortunately, all our information on wife assaults arises from retrospective reconstructions from a highly select sample. Women in the Rounsaville and the

Rosenbaum and O'Leary studies came only from emergency wards and shelters. Because only 8.6% of assaults are reported to police (Schulman, 1980) and they act on only half of these (Levens & Dutton, 1977), any reconstructions based on police cases can also be highly unrepresentative. Essentially, the problem in the prediction of wife assault is that an especially large *chiffe noire* precludes the possibility of acquiring requisite baseline data. Even the seemingly high incidence of violence in the family of origin may not differ significantly from baseline rates for nonassaultive men when substantial data for the latter group become available. If this is the case, the weight given to this factor in the etiology of wife assault may shrink. Until such data are available, prediction is precarious and the risk of a substantial number of false positives is great.

Notes

1 For the purposes of this chapter, the term "wife" refers to all women in intimate relationships with the assaultive man, regardless of legal marital status. "Assault" refers to the physical expression of male dominance over women.
2 This estimate was based on the conservative assumption that there was no underreporting due to "image management."

References

Bandura, A. *Aggression: A sound-learning analysis.* Englewood Cliffs, N.J.: Prentice-Hall, 1973.
Belsky, J. Child maltreatment: An ecological integration. *American Psychologist,* 1980, *35,* 320–35.
Burt, M. Cultural myths and support for rape. *Journal of Personality and Social Psychology,* 1980, *38*(2), 217–30.
Curley, A. D., & O'Leary, K. J. *Psychological correlates of spouse abuse.* Paper presented at the American Association for Behavior Therapy, New York, N.Y., November 21, 1980.
Davidson, T. Wifebeating: A recurring phenomenon throughout history. In M. Roy (Ed.), *Battered women: A psychological study of domestic violence.* New York: Van Nostrand, 1977.
de Reincourt, A. *Sex and power in history.* New York: Delta, 1974.
Diagnostic and statistical manual of the mental disorders (3rd ed.). Washington, D.C.: American Psychiatric Association, 1980.
Dobash, R. E., & Dobash, R. *Violence against wives.* New York: Free Press, 1979.
Dutton, D. G. Issues in domestic crisis intervention programmer for police. In *Family violence.* Symposium presented by United Way of Greater Vancouver, 1977.
Dutton, D. G. Training police officers to intervene in domestic violence. In R. Stuart (Ed.), *Violent behavior: Social learning approaches.* New York: Brunner/Mazel, 1981.
Dutton, D. G. *The criminal justice system response to wife assault.* Ottawa: Solicitor General of Canada, 1982.
Dutton, D. G. An ecologically nested theory of male violence toward intimates. In P. Caplan (Ed.), *Sex Roles* (Vol. 2), *Feminist psychology in transition.* Montreal: Eden Press, 1984.
Dutton, D. G., Fehr, B., & McEwen, H. Severe wife battering as deindividuated violence. *Victimology,* 1982, *7,* 13–23.
Dutton, D. G., & Painter, S. L. Male domestic violence and its effects on the victim. Ottawa: Health and Welfare, 1980.

Dutton, D. G., & Painter, S. L. Traumatic bonding: The development of emotional attachments in battered women and other relationships of intermittent abuse. *Victimology*, 1981, *6*, 139–55.

Elbow, M. Theoretical considerations of violent marriages. *Social Casework*, November 1977, pp. 515–26.

Ganley, A., & Harris, L. *Domestic violence: Issues in designing and implementing programmes for male batterers.* Paper presented at the American Psychological Association, Toronto, 1978.

Gelles, R. J. *The violent home: A study of physical aggression between husbands and wives.* Beverly Hills: Sage, 1974.

Gelles, R. Violence and pregnancy: A note on the extent of the problem and needed services. *The Family Co-ordinator*, 1975, *24*, 81–6.

Heale, W. An apology for women: That it was lawful for husbands to beat their wives (1609). In M. Roy (Ed.), *Battered women: A psychosocial study of domestic violence.* New York: Van Nostrand, 1977.

Hunt, M. *The natural history of love.* New York: Knopf, 1959.

Jaffe, P. Testimony before Standing Committee on Health, Welfare, and Social Affairs. House of Commons, Ottawa, February 11, 1982, p. 27:15.

Kramer, H., & Sprenger, J. *Malleus maleficarum* (M. Summers, trans.). New York: Oxford University Press, 1928. (Original publication, 1484.)

Levens, B., & Dutton, D. Domestic crisis intervention: Citizens' requests for service and the Vancouver Police Department response. *Canadian Police College Journal*, 1977, *1*, 50.

Levens, B. R., & Dutton, D. G. *The social service role of the police: Domestic crisis intervention.* Ottawa: Solicitor General of Canada, 1980.

Martin, D. *Battered wives.* New York: Kangaroo Paperbacks, 1977.

McClelland, D. *Power: The inner experience.* New York: Halsted Press, 1975.

Meichenbaum, D. *Cognitive behavior modification.* Morristown, N.J.: General Learning Press, 1974.

Metzger, M. *A social history of battered women.* Ottawa: Secretary of State, Multiculturalism, 1980.

Mill, J. S. *The subjection of women* (1869) (Introduction by W. R. Carr), Cambridge, Mass.: M.I.T. Press, 1970.

Novaco, R. *Anger control: The development and evaluation of an experimental treatment.* Lexington, Mass.: Lexington Books, 1975.

Novaco, R. The functions and regulation of the arousal of anger. *American Journal of Psychiatry*, 1976, *122*, 11–28.

Parnas, R. I. Prosecutorial and judicial handling of family violence. *Criminal Law Bulletin*, 1973, *9*, 733.

Patterson, M. L. An arousal model of interpersonal intimacy. *Psychological Review*, 1976, *83*(3), 235–45.

Rathus, S. A. A 30-item schedule for assessing assertive behavior. *Behavior Therapy*, 1973, *4*, 498–506.

Rosenbaum, A., & O'Leary, K. D. Marital violence. *Journal of Consulting and Clinical Psychology*, 1981, *41*, 63.

Rounsaville, B. Theories in marital violence: Evidence from a study of battered women. *Victimology*, 1978, *3*, 11–31.

Ryan, W. *Blaming the victim.* New York: Vintage, 1971.

Schulman, M. *A survey of spousal violence against women in Kentucky.* Washington, D.C.: U.S. Department of Justice, Law Enforcement Assistance and Administration, 1980.

Shotland, L., & Straw, M. Bystander response to an assault: When a man attacks a woman. *Journal of Personality and Social Psychology*, 1976, *34*, 990–9.

Sommer, R. *Personal space: The behavioral basis of design.* Englewood Cliffs, N.J.: Prentice-Hall, 1969.

Stark, R., & McEvoy, J. Middle class violence. *Psychology Today*, 1970, *4*, 107–112.

Steinmetz, S., & Straus, M. (Eds.) *Violence in the family.* New York: Harper & Row, 1974.

Straus, M. A general systems theory approach to a theory of violence between family members. *Social Science Information,* 1973, *12,* 105–25.

Straus, M. A. Sexual inequality, cultural norm and wife beating. *Victimology,* 1976, *1,* 54–76.

Straus, M. A. Societal morphogenesis and intrafamily violence in cross-cultural perspective. *Annals of the New York Academy of Sciences,* 1977, *285,* 718–30. (a)

Straus, M. Violence in the family: How widespread, why it occurs and some thoughts on prevention. In *Family violence,* Symposium presented by United Way of Greater Vancouver, 1977. (b)

Straus, M., Gelles, R. J., & Steinmetz, S. K. *Behind closed doors: Violence in the American family.* New York: Anchor Books, 1980.

Symonds, M. The Psychodynamics of violence-prone marriages. *American Journal of Psychoanalysis,* 1978, *38,* 213.

Szinovacz, M. Using couple data as a methodological tool: The case of marital violence. *Journal of Marriage and the Family,* August 1983, pp. 633–44.

Taylor, G. R. *Sex in history.* New York: Vanguard Press, 1954.

U.S. Commission on Civil Rights. *Battered women: Issues of public policy.* Washington, D.C.: U.S. Government Printing Office, 1978.

Whitehurst, R. N. Violence in husband – wife interaction. In S. Steinmetz & M. Straus (Eds.), *Violence in the family.* New York: Harper & Row, 1974.

Wilt, G. M., & Breedlove, R. K. *Domestic violence and the police: studies in Detroit and Kansas City.* Washington, D.C.: Police Foundation, 1977.

Winter, D. G. *The power motive.* New York: Free Press, 1973.

Zimbardo, P. The human choice: Individuation, reason and order vs. deindividuation, impulse and chaos. In W. J. Arnold & D. Levine (Eds.), *Nebraska Symposium on Motivation* (Vol. 17). Lincoln: University of Nebraska Press, 1969.

8   Hitting the forensic sound barrier: predictions of dangerousness in a pretrial psychiatric clinic

Robert J. Menzies, Christopher D. Webster,
and Diana S. Sepejak

Life is the art of drawing sufficient conclusions from insufficient premises.
Samuel Butler, *Notebooks Life IX*

Science is what we know, and philosophy is what we don't know.
Bertrand Russell, *Unpopular Essays* (1950)

Introduction: The criminology and psychiatry of dangerousness

Social and behavioral scientists work with the materials of probability. In contrast to the objectivity of the natural sciences, value judgments, normative assumptions, and decision making under conditions of doubt are constants in social research and policy. Claims of objectivity and disinterest have long been discredited as so much positivistic mystification. The fact is that social scientists and practitioners are burdened with the subjectivity of their own interests, beliefs, and affiliations (Brown, 1977; Cunningham, 1973). To deny these influences is to construct a false image of professionalism and expertise, which is belied by the history of our enterprise.

Nowhere is this principle more applicable than in the area of criminal justice decision making. The development of positive criminology in the late nineteenth and early twentieth centuries was based on speculation that universal laws of behavior were discoverable, that criminology could operate on the natural sciences model, and – most crucially – that researchers and official decision makers

This research was funded primarily by the Ontario Ministry of Health under Grant DM395. Additional support came from the Department of Justice, Canada, and the Law Foundation of Ontario and was indirectly facilitated by the Ministry of the Solicitor General, Canada's contribution program to the Centre of Criminology, University of Toronto. Thanks to Roy Gillis and Val Cattelan for their research assistance.

115

could, with the instruments of science, construct their systems of justice and policy around the predicted criminality of individuals (Mannheim, 1960; Rennie, 1978; Taylor, Walton, & Young, 1973; Vold, 1958). The confidence in the predictive capacity of officials has had a profound impact, to the present day, on systems of preventive detention and individualization of punishment (Rothman, 1980; von Hirsch, 1976). As Monahan (1981) has written, "Prediction has always been a part of life and has always been a part of law" (p. 6).

This chapter concerns itself with the prediction of dangerousness by psychiatric professionals. Since the mid-1960s, the construct of dangerousness and its attribution by forensic experts have acquired a high profile in the fields of criminology and psychiatry (Hamilton & Freeman, 1982; Hinton, 1983; Monahan, 1981; Pfohl, 1978; Rappeport, 1967; Steadman & Cocozza, 1974; Thornberry & Jacoby, 1979; Van Dine, Conrad, & Dinitz, 1979). The ascent of the dangerousness controversy has been marked by a fundamental irony of intention and result. On the one hand, standards of dangerousness in civil commitment (Boyd, 1980; Dershowitz, 1969; Hiday, 1981; Schrieber, 1970; Shah, 1975), dangerous offender legislation (Klein, 1976; Price, 1970), and the release of institutionalized subjects (Gunn, Robertson, & Way, 1978; Lipton, Martinson, & Wilks, 1975; Morris, 1974; Rappeport, 1967; Steadman & Cocozza, 1974; Thornberry and Jacoby, 1979) have emerged from an essentially humanitarian philosophy: "The contemporary concern with identifying and isolating dangerous people appears tied to liberal or reformist movements within mental health and criminal justice circles, with efforts to secure rights for the involuntarily institutionalized through depopulating mental hospitals and prisons of all but those who are 'truly' dangerous" (Pfohl, 1979, p. 55). On the other hand, civil libertarians have uniformly attacked a medicolegal system that confines and retains individuals on the basis of anticipated future violence: "In the case of decisions about possible dangerousness, heuristics lead systematically to a 'public protectionist' model based on conservative clinical decisions producing many false positives and fewer false negatives. Typically, errors of the false positive type are unseen as they are tucked away unnecessarily in maximum security hospitals or special security units" (Steadman & Morrissey, 1981, p. 273).

The literature on the prediction of dangerousness during the past decade has been legion (Floud & Young, 1982; Hamilton & Freeman, 1982; Hinton, 1983; Monahan, 1981; Pfohl, 1978). Three fundamental themes permeate this research. First, dangerousness is an ephemeral concept that is repeatedly confounded by such related constructs as psychopathy, violence, assaultiveness, dangerous *behavior,* and criminality. As Sarbin (1967) wrote in his seminal article, dangerousness is essentially a *relationship,* which varies not only with behavior, but according to institutional context, interpretive processes, and social reaction. "Dangerousness can be so loosely interpreted as to include any behavior, physical appearance, or mental condition stated to be dangerous" (Hiday & Markell, 1980, p. 416).

Second, the prediction of dangerousness is not only a clinical pursuit, but also an exercise in legal control with political overtones (Petrunik, 1983; Rennie, 1978; Warren, 1979). Wenk, Robison, & Smith (1978) write that "confidence in the ability to predict violence serves to legitimate intrusive types of social control" (p. 402). Rennie (1978) contends that " 'dangerous offender' is a protean concept, changing its color and shape to suit the fears, interests, needs and prejudices of a society. . . . It is an *idea,* not a person" (p. 17).

Third, psychiatrists have been found incapable of predicting dangerousness with any degree of reliability or accuracy. Errors systematically load in the direction of overprediction of violence (Ennis & Litwack, 1974; Steadman & Cocozza, 1974; Thornberry & Jacoby, 1979). Heuristic entanglements native to low base-rate predictions have been extensively discussed in both the general psychological (Bem & Allen, 1974; Bem & Funder, 1978; Mischel, 1968; Sawyer, 1966; Wiggins, 1973) and forensic literature (Monahan, 1981; Quinsey, 1980; Rubin, 1972; Shah, 1978; Steadman, 1976). Moreover, forensic prognostics fail to take account of the context-bound situationality of dangerous behavior. For instance, Levinson and Ramsay (1979) found that situational stress is a fairly reliable index of dangerousness. A multitude of contextual factors, subsequent to prediction, can shape and redirect the course of an individual's violent career. Megargee (1976) has enumerated some of these: "the availability of a weapon, the presence of onlookers, and the behaviour of a potential victim, but [also] more pervasive situational variables such as the level of frustration in the environment, or the social approval of violence in a particular subculture" (p. 9).

The majority of prediction research is based on follow-ups of patients released from psychiatric institutions (e.g., Dix, 1975; Kozol, Boucher, & Garafolo, 1972; Quinsey et al., 1975; Steadman & Cocozza, 1974; Thornberry & Jacoby, 1979). Although these studies demonstrate an absence of predictive skills on the part of clinicians, a number of conceptual and methodological problems are inherent in such studies. The selective nature of subject populations mitigates the generalizability of these findings. Furthermore, this research is notably lacking in efforts to analyze the clinical decision-making process, preventing the documentation and measurement of component judgments underlying predictions. Kozol et al. (1972) discuss general areas of inquiry explored by clinicians, but judgments in these areas were not measured and compared with the final opinion. Dix (1975) observed the deliberations of a clinical team deciding on the dangerousness of committed patients but failed to gauge the prognostic power of principles extracted from these discussions. In the most rigorous study to date of dangerousness decisions, Pfohl (1978) extensively documented the cognitive and interpersonal strategies of multidisciplinary teams but did not validate their accuracy through the use of outcome data.

With Monahan (1981), we argue that methodological flaws in the current literature belie the conclusory language in which much of the discussion is couched. In a real sense, the jury is still out on the empirical question of prediction–outcome associations. This observation does *not* necessarily prejudice the ethical, legal, and sociolegal implications of dangerousness prediction (see Bottoms, 1977). There is an argument that, even in the unlikely event that technological innovation could yield perfect predictive accuracy, dangerousness would remain a "dangerous concept" (Scott, 1977, p. 127). These are social policy issues, which must be combined with empirical research to bring resolutions to the dangerousness problem.

Before turning to our own research on predictions of dangerousness, we shall outline our criteria for an "ideal study" in this area. These standards can be invoked to assess the limitations of the present study, as well as others in the dangerousness literature. The following criteria are essential for maximum internal and external validity:

1. The sample should be neither self-selected nor institutionally assigned.
2. The research should not interfere with the ordinary clinical process.
3. Subjects should be controlled or matched across critical psychiatric and sociological variables.
4. Clinicians should have an opportunity to influence the format in which predictions are expressed.
5. Predictions should be continuous rather than dichotomous, and free-form rather than forced-choice.
6. The patient's psychosocial environment should be incorporated into the decision-making dynamic.
7. Multiple professions and individuals must be involved in making predictions.
8. These clinicians should render *independent* decisions, and patients should be *randomly* assigned to individual assessors and groups.
9. All terms and definitions should be rigorously operationalized.
10. Predictions of nondangerousness as well as dangerousness should be available to clinicians.
11. The degree of certainty should be indicated along with the prediction.
12. There must be both quantitative and qualitative analysis of the decision-making process, predictions made individually being compared with group ratings.
13. Inter-rater reliability should be measured; to the degree possible, there should be no systematic differences in outcome conditions among patients at different levels of predicted dangerousness.
14. Measures of outcome should be triangulated, employing both official data and self-report instruments, in the community, justice, and mental health systems.
15. Length of follow-up should be at least 3 years and equal for all subjects; instruments should gauge both short-term and protracted dangerousness.
16. The relationship between prediction and outcome should be analyzed on both relative (covariation) and absolute associations (level).

METFORS dangerousness research

Clinical context

Metropolitan Toronto Forensic Service (METFORS) was opened in September 1977. METFORS is situated in a Canadian city of 2.5 million people; it is funded principally by the provincial attorney general and administered through the Clarke Institute of Psychiatry. The Brief Assessment Unit (BAU) of METFORS began operation on January 23, 1978. The BAU is designed to provide 1-day forensic assessments, under maximum-security conditions, of accused individuals before the criminal courts in Metropolitan Toronto. The major innovation of the BAU is the multidisciplinary nature of the assessment process. Patients undergoing assessment are interviewed by a clinical team comprising a psychiatrist, psychologist, social worker, forensic nurse, and correctional officer (see Butler & Turner, 1980; Webster, Menzies, & Jackson, 1982).

On a typical working day, two to four individuals receive evaluation and are returned to the local detention center in the afternoon accompanied by a letter dictated by the psychiatrist and addressed to the presiding judge. About one-fourth of the patients are remanded for protracted assessment, a few are referred for 30 to 60 days to another psychiatric unit, and occasionally individuals are certified under provincial mental health legislation. The primary concern of the BAU team is generally fitness to stand trial (see McGarry et al., 1973; Roesch & Golding, 1980; Webster et al., 1982). Contingent on the nature of the case and inquiries directed to the clinic by the court, the mental health team may address such discretionary issues as general mental status, treatability, recommended disposition, and dangerousness to self and/or others.

BAU patients

From the opening of the BAU to the end of 1978, 665 forensic assessments were conducted. Of these, 67 were second or third assessments of the same person; for the purposes of the dangerousness study, these multiple remands were deleted, leaving a sample size of 598.

The characteristics of pretrial forensic populations have been discussed elsewhere in great detail (e.g., Gibbens, Soothill, & Pope, 1977; Greenland & Rosenblatt, 1972; Laczko, James, & Alltop 1970; Pfeiffer, Eisenstein, & Dabbs, 1967; Roesch & Golding, 1980). The general impression gained from this research is that of a patient cohort heterogeneous in both legal and psychosocial background. Criminal charges range from loitering to first-degree murder; level of pathology from normality to paranoid schizophrenia. The common denominator in such populations is the individuals' consistently peripheral and disenfranchised socioeconomic condition. These are the semiinstitutionalized groups described by Scull (1977), Bassuk and Gerson (1978), Segal and Aviram (1978), and others, who are subject to the interlocking controls of welfare, justice, and mental health and whose deviant careers penetrate repeatedly into these three systems of supervision and restraint.

The METFORS patients displayed behavior and histories characteristic of marginal clientele. Of 598 patients, 537 were men. Forty-nine percent had been previously incarcerated; only 20% had no previous involvement with the criminal courts. Fifty-one percent had been hospitalized in a psychiatric institution; one-third were diagnosed as having personality disorders and one-fourth as psychotic. Of 504 patients for whom data were available, 130 (26%) had no more than grade-school education. Thirty-two percent were unemployed at the time of arrest. Fifty percent consumed alcohol excessively; 30% were heavy abusers of other drugs.

Dangerousness decisions: Sources of independent variables

The clinical assessments were derived from two sources: (a) one-page instrument schedules completed by BAU members for research purposes and (b) the medical records and court letters written by the forensic team. About one-third of psychiatric letters to the court specifically address the issue of dangerousness (Henderson, 1980); in this study, the patients' medical records are used primarily for illustrative purposes (see case histories given later). The assessment instruments, in contrast, comprise the primary index of dangerousness decisions.[1] Along with a number of other forced-choice decisions, psychiatrists and other clinicians were asked to rate the following for each subject: present dangerousness to self, present dangerousness to others, future dangerousness to self, and future dangerousness to others. These judgments were recorded on a four-point scale (1, no; 2, low; 3, medium; 4, high); clinicians indicated "unclear" if no decision could be reached. The BAU team members were instructed to complete their ratings immediately after the interview and before discussing the case among themselves; although we are reasonably confident about the independence of the ratings, it is impossible to judge the degree to which mutual accommodation and convergence of impressions may develop during the interview itself (see Pfohl, 1978, 1979). The composition of the team changed on a day-to-day basis; in all, 4 psychiatrists, 2 psychiatric residents, 4 psychologists, 3 social workers, 5 nurses, and 14 correctional officers were involved in evaluating the 598 cases during 1978. It is important to note that the participants, like the researchers themselves, had no idea that the predictions would eventually be checked. The possibility presented itself long after the data had been collected and stored.

This study was concerned with predictions of dangerousness (i.e., to others in

Table 8.1. *Distributions of dangerousness predictions for five professional groups*

Professional group	N	Percentage of no danger (1)	Percentage of low danger (2)	Percentage of medium danger (3)	Percentage of high danger (4)	$\bar{X}$	SD	Number of "unclear" decisions	Member not present
Psychiatrists	516	15.7	33.4	34.8	16.1	2.51	0.94	72	11
Psychologists	410	13.4	21.7	37.6	27.3	2.79	0.99	81	107
Social workers	392	7.7	32.1	31.9	28.3	2.81	0.94	36	170
Nurses	450	27.8	16.0	32.4	23.8	2.52	1.13	108	40
Correctional officers	384	20.8	17.2	33.1	28.9	2.70	1.10	166	48

the future). It would appear, first, that dangerousness predictions on the four-point scale are quite reliable across the five clinical groups. For example, Table 8.1 illustrates that average predictions for the five professions are of similar magnitude. Social workers indicated the highest mean dangerousness for patients ($\bar{X} = 2.81$), whereas psychiatrists indicated the lowest ($\bar{X} = 2.51$). In addition, it was possible to gauge inter-rater reliability by generating a kappa statistic for cases evaluated by all five professions ($n = 151$). This exhibited a significant level of inter-rater agreement (kappa = .26, SD = .017, $Z = 15.53$, $p < .001$).

Dangerousness outcomes: Establishing a criterion

As Monahan has argued (1981), relating the concept of dangerousness to specific behavioral indicators presents an intransigent obstacle for dangerousness research. Such outcome measures as assaultiveness (Steadman & Cocozza, 1978), personal offenses (Hodges, 1971), violent violations of parole (Wenk et al., 1972), and self-reports of violent behavior (Thornberry & Jacoby, 1979) have been used as dependent variables in previous studies. Several difficulties are inherent in these and other projects (Monahan, 1981). First, few attempts have been made to triangulate follow-up assaultiveness by concatenating official data, self-reports, and victimization analysis. Second, the majority of longitudinal traces of violence have been limited to police records or criminal justice data. This oversight produces "grossly truncated measures" (Hall, 1982, p. 6), which are insensitive to both the dark figure of undetected violence and assaultiveness occurring in mental health in addition to criminal justice institutions. Third, the length of follow-up is a critical determinant of violence potential; studies that employ varying longitudinal time frames (e.g., Kozol et al., 1972) are vulnerable to systematic distortions in outcome data. Fourth, the courses of subsequent patient careers are usually dependent to a degree on the predictions themselves. This consideration may bias prediction–outcome associations in two ways. The attribution of dangerousness may function as a self-fulfilling prophecy (Holland, 1979; Pfohl, 1978; Warren, 1979), solidifying the subject's self-conception as a dangerous person and amplifying the career of violence. Alternatively, predictions of violence may reinforce the probability of confinement, thereby decreasing the environmental opportunity for assaultive behavior and attenuating the demonstrated relation between prediction and outcome. Fifth, most studies lack external validity, in that subjects are typically discharged from prisons (Gunn et al., 1978; Ribner & Steadman, 1981; Waller, 1974), security hospitals (Quinsey et al., 1975; Steadman & Cocozza, 1974; Thornberry & Jacoby, 1979), or general psychiatric institutions (Giovannoni & Gurel, 1967; Guze, Woodruff, & Clayton, 1974; Mesnikoff & Lauterbach, 1975; Sasowsky, 1978; Zitrin, Hardesty, Burdock, & Drosaman, 1976).

The design of the present study and the outcome measure employed in the follow-up are subject, as in other research, to several of these deficiencies. Conversely, some difficulties have been remedied. Each of the 598 patients was followed up for 2 years after his or her BAU assessment. Two sources of data were used. First, 24 months after assessment, the Ontario Ministry of Correctional Services Central Registry was reviewed for evidence of contact with each subject. Second, the records of six major psychiatric hospitals in the southern Ontario region were consulted to determine the incidence of dangerous behavior leading to or occurring during mental institutionalization. Four categories of outcome incidents were compiled: criminal convictions, misconducts during incarceration, reasons for contact with hospital, and behavior during hospital contact.

All charges, misconducts, and incidents during the 24 months were aggregated for each patient.[2] At least one entry was recorded for 408 subjects (68%).[3] Altogether, these 408 individuals, over 24 months, were involved in 1,219 criminal charges, 548 misconducts during incarceration, 327 incidents leading to psychiatric hospital contact, and 329 in-hospital record entries. A flow chart outlining the channeling of subjects is provided in Figure 8.1.

After considerable debate, we decided to exclude from further analysis those 190 cases for whom no follow-up records were recovered. We did this for two reasons. First, it is impossible to ascertain whether an absence of a follow-up record signifies the nonexistence of incidents or merely the failure of official systems to detect the subject's activities. The strong coincidence, in many cases, of missing data for both "court disposition" and "outcome" lends support to the latter hypothesis. Second, in the development of the ratio scale of outcome dangerousness discussed later, it could not be established that a difference between a "no" response and a score of 1 was equivalent to the difference between any other two adjacent scores.[4]

For each of the 408 cases, a summary was constructed that enumerated all incidents in which the subject was involved under the four conditions. These

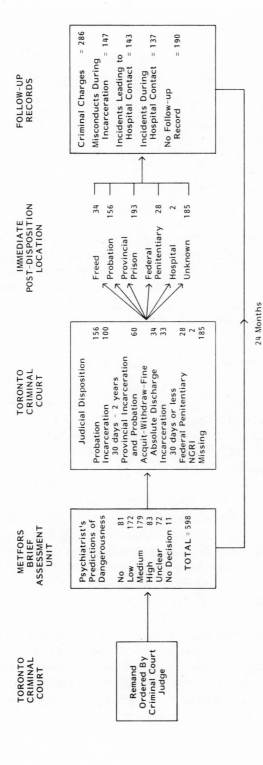

Figure 8.1. Flow chart showing how subjects were channeled during the two-year follow-up period (NGRI = not guilty by reason of insanity).

Table 8.2. *Dangerousness Outcome Scores (DOS) distribution*

	DOS								
	1	2	3	4	5	6	7	8	9
N	14	84	68	59	77	60	37	7	2
Percentage	3.4	20.6	16.7	14.5	18.9	14.7	9.1	1.7	0.5

Note: Missing cases = 190.

outcomes were quantified on dangerousness through the use of independent judges. Three MA-level criminology students rated each case summary for dangerousness to others on a scale of 1 to 11.[5] On analysis, inter-rater reliability among the three judges reached acceptable levels.[6] The scores for the three judges were then averaged and integerized to generate a Dangerousness Outcome Score (DOS) for all 408 patients.[7] Mean DOS was 4.17. Table 8.2 presents the distribution of DOS scores for the sample, and Table 8.3 exhibits a typical case summary located at each of the nine DOS levels.

Results 1: Relationship between patient background and outcome danger

The prediction of dangerousness from objective indicators represents what Gottfredson (1971) has termed a "narrow band" process of decision making. Actuarial models (Wenk et al., 1972) and quantitative scores based on legal criteria (Steadman & Cocozza, 1974) have been singularly unproductive in refining forensic prognostics concerning violence. As Hall (1982) writes, "It is no surprise that correlation coefficients of subject characteristics and later violence have not exceeded the .40 'sound barrier', despite adding a multitude of information to the prediction equation or clinical judgment process" (p. 5). Forensic professionals apparently vary in the number and weight of different legal/psychiatric variables that they consider when deciding on dangerousness (Pfohl, 1979). At the same time, a history of violent behavior has been demonstrated by several observers (e.g., Monahan, 1981; Steadman & Cocozza, 1974) to be the best single "objective" indicator of future dangerousness. It is clear that the probability of assaultiveness increases with each past act of violence (Shah, 1978; Wolfgang, 1978). Yet such exploratory findings have been neither effectively actuarialized nor embedded into clinical decision making. As a result, there is a tendency for objective factors and intuitional judgments to be mutually nugatory rather than reinforcing. In fact, Diamond (1974) suggests that reference to objective criteria may legitimate an erroneous decision-making process: "It would be difficult for an objective observer to take such claims seriously if such pseudo-

Table 8.3. *Sample follow-up dangerousness scores*

Score	Case number	Criminal charges	Misconducts during incarceration	Reason for contact with hospital	Behavior during hospital contact
1	427	—	—	Spent 3 days sitting on street corner	—
2	095	Theft under $200 (×2), municipal bylaws (×2), willful non-compliance with terms of bail or probation, breach of highway traffic act	Neglected performing the work or duty assigned to him	—	—
3	336	—	—	Angry and hostile, depressed and upset because he is unable to obtain welfare and has no place to stay, generally depressed, dissatisfied with present lodgings	Easily angered, afraid of others, left hospital twice without being formally discharged
4	201	—	Caused or threatened to cause a disturbance or riot, attacked or threatened to attack another person in the institution, had in his possession unauthorized articles, conducted himself in a manner detrimental to other inmates or to the institutional program	—	—
5	469	Mischief, possession under $200, unlawfully in dwelling house, harassment (×2), false news (×2)	Had contraband in his possession or participated in an attempt to bring contraband in or take contraband out of the institution	Threatened someone, threatened to choke mother, argumentative	Negativistic, obscene, assaulted staff, pacing excessively, verbally and physically abusive, threatened to kick staff in head
6	334	—	—	Depressed, problems looking after himself	Hostile and angry, threatened to kill copatient, pointed finger in threatening manner at nurse

Table 8.3. (cont.)

Score	Case number	Criminal charges	Misconducts during incarceration	Reason for contact with hospital	Behavior during hospital contact
7	513	Bodily assault	—	—	Threatened staff and copatients with bodily harm, threw urine at staff, threatened staff with bodily harm, threatened to kill a copatient, threatened and spit at staff, banging doors and screaming
8	022	Procuring, fraud involving transportation, escape, common assault	Attacked or threatened to attack another person within the institution (×3)	—	Struck copatient, suddenly attacked copatient, delivering several blows to head and causing bleeding, struck copatient a blow to left side of head, attacked attendant, tried on numerous occasions to kick and punch staff, punched attendant in eye, struck copatient in face and chest, struck copatient, struck copatient a blow to right side of head
9	590	Trafficking in narcotics, assault causing bodily harm	Willfully disobeyed a lawful order of an officer, committed or threatened to commit an assault on another person	Hearing voices say terrible things about him and his family, overdosed on drugs, attempted suicide, mumbling to himself, threatened younger brother with an ax following an overdose of drugs while drinking beer, hearing voices talking to him about snakes and committing suicide, inappropriate giggling and smiling, smashed up mother's apartment and attempted to strangle her with a cord, alcohol abuse	Gross thought disorder, sarcastic, seclusive, preoccupied with voices

scientific descriptions had not been reiterated so often that they had become part of the accepted mythology of clinical practice'' (p. 443; see also Pfohl, 1978).

In the present study, we undertook to examine the discriminating power of background variables on the DOS. Nineteen patient characteristics were subjected to difference of means tests, with DOS ratings as the dependent variable. (These variables were of five general classes: sociodemographic, legal, psychiatric, socioeconomic, and alcohol/drug use.) Only four variables significantly differentiated DOS means (Table 8.4).There were no differences among sociodemographic or economic categories of patients (e.g., age, gender, occupation, and education) in follow-up levels of dangerousness. Legal history, however, achieved some discriminatory power. Those with a history of violent offenses and with previous time spent in prison were more dangerous than others during the 24-month follow-up. The nature of the current charge (violent or nonviolent) failed to yield significantly different means. It is interesting that the 179 patients with a record of psychiatric hospitalization were significantly *less* dangerous than those without such histories. Finally, higher average DOS ratings were obtained for those individuals who were perceived to be hostile or delusional during the initial assessment.

The marginal mean differences realized by these bivariate procedures exhibit little predictive utility. Accordingly, we set out to determine the *maximum possible* predictive power obtainable from these background variables. The DOS ratings were dichotomized by median, and a multiple discriminant analysis was run on 16 independent variables.[8] Bayesian corrections were made for prior probabilities (59% were ''nondangerous'' on follow-up). The results are summarized in Table 8.5.

Using a multivariate framework for analysis, one finds that the four factors with the highest relative discriminating power are attitude/behavior when assessed, alcohol use, previous incarceration, and age. When the dangerousness of subjects is predicted according to the best possible weighting of actuarial factors, 63.7% of cases are correctly classified. This amounts to only a 4% improvement over base-rate predictions (i.e., that 41% would be dangerous). The ratio of false positives to true positives is approximately 3:2; of those that are above the median DOS of 4.14, only slightly more than one/half are correctly predicted. These results lend further credence to Megargee's (1970) observation 15 years ago that no methods have been devised ''which will adequately *post*-dict, let alone *pre*dict, violent behavior'' (p. 145).

Results 2: Clinical predictions and follow-up dangerousness

The level of association between clinical prediction and DOS ratings was measured for all professional groups. To the extent that diagnoses of dangerousness

Table 8.4. *Difference of means tests: background variables and Dangerousness Outcome Score*

Background variable	t	df	p	Group 1			Group 2		
				N	$\bar{X}$	SE	N	$\bar{X}$	SE
History of violent offenses	−1.98	368	.05	Nonviolent (190)	4.02	.13	Violent (180)	4.39	.14
Previous incarceration	−2.70	358	.007	No (164)	3.93	.15	Yes (196)	4.46	.13
Previous hospitalization	2.18	328	.03	No (179)	4.27	.13	Yes (151)	3.84	.15
Attitude and behavior during assessment (hostile, acting out, or delusional?)	−2.26	362	.03	No (150)	3.94	.15	Yes (214)	4.38	.13

Table 8.5. *Multiple discriminant analysis: dangerousness during 24-month follow-up*

Bayesian prior probabilities		Independent variable	Standardized discriminant function coefficient
Nondangerous	.59	Attitude/behavior when assessed	.59
Dangerous	.41	Alcohol use	−.56
		Previous incarceration	.45
Group centroids		Age (dichotomized at 30 years)	.44
Nondangerous	−.32	Previous involvement with law	.41
Dangerous	.46	Previous hospitalization?	.40
		Violent charge?	.37
Wilks' lambda	87	Gender	−.29

$(\chi^2 = 19.74, df = 8, p = .01)$

Actual dangerousness	Predicted dangerousness		
	Low	High	Total
Low	83	31	114
	(66.4%)	(40.8%)	
High	42	45	87
	(33.6%)	(59.2%)	
Total	125	76	201

are clinical rather than legal categories, we would expect psychiatrists to fare better than other professionals. This hypothesis was moderately borne out by the data. Psychiatrists as a group achieved a .20 zero-order correlation compared with .17 for psychologists and .12 or less for members of the other mental health disciplines (Table 8.6). It is also noteworthy that considerable intergroup variations in predictive accuracy were obtained. The correlations for all clinicians who rated 10 or more patients with DOS scores are presented in Table 8.6.

Individual psychiatrists' accuracies ranged from .03 to .27, those of psychologists from .14 to .21, those of social workers from .02 to .47, those of nurses from .10 to .29, and those of correctional officers from − .48 to .23. Although these generally positive findings may seem encouraging, two major limitations should be noted. First, Pearson correlations do not measure the *absolute* accuracy of prediction levels (i.e., no, low, medium, and high), but only *relative* covariation of prediction and outcome (see R. B. Haynes, chapter 4). Second, the proportion of follow-up variance accounted for by predictions was minimal. Even social worker 3, the sole clinician to break the .40 "sound barrier," could anticipate only 22% of the variance in her predictions.

Another relevant consideration is raised by P. E. Dietz in chapter 6: It may be that some forensic patients are more predictable than others, that is, that an interaction effect between clinician and subject may shape accuracy rates. Sev-

Table 8.6. *Prediction–outcome correlations:*
dangerousness to others

Predictor	r^a	n	p
All psychiatrists	.20	364	.001[b]
Psychiatrist 1	.19	160	.009[b]
Psychiatrist 2	.14	75	.112
Psychiatrist 3	.27	86	.006[b]
Psychiatrist 4	.03	43	.415
All psychologists	.17	288	.002[b]
Psychologist 1	.21	137	.007[b]
Psychologist 2	.21	67	.043[b]
Psychologist 3	.14	68	.134
All social workers	.03	273	.301
Social worker 1	.02	224	.402
Social worker 2	.12	16	.332
Social worker 3	.47	16	.032[b]
All nurses	.08	309	.069
Nurse 1	.10	264	.046[b]
Nurse 2	.29	23	.087
All correctional officers	.12	266	.030[b]
Correctional officer 1	.21	13	.244
Correctional officer 2	.22	28	.127
Correctional officer 3	−.48	10	.079
Correctional officer 4	.23	31	.106
Correctional officer 5	.04	48	.388
Correctional officer 6	.07	38	.341
Correctional officer 7	.20	42	.092

[a] Pearson product–moment correlations between prediction of dangerousness to others and dangerousness outcome score.
[b] $p < .05$.

eral commentators have argued that only those individuals with a history of psychopathy or violence should be subject to dangerousness determinations. Megargee (1976) writes, "Mental health professionals should limit themselves to predicting dangerous behavior in high base-rate populations such as those who have already engaged in repeated violence" (p. 18).

We examined the variations in predictive accuracy for psychiatrists across patients with different records of violence and mental disorder. Different patterns emerge for each of the four psychiatrists. Psychiatrist 1's prediction–outcome correlations did not vary substantially for the three patient diagnoses used (psychosis, personality disorder, and other); he was, however, more accurate in assessing patients charged with a nonviolent offence ($r = .23$) than those arrested

Table 8.7. *"Hits" and "misses" for clinician groups*

Clinicians	False positives	Low hits	False negatives	High hits
Psychiatrists	61	86	15	27
Psychologists	78	45	9	26
Social workers	59	40	12	18
Nurses	59	61	12	22
Correctional officers	58	40	9	26

for a violent incident ($r = .09$). Psychiatrist 2 was unable to predict patients with a charge of violence ($r = -.15$) or "other" diagnoses ($r = -.19$); he was considerably more accurate with nonviolent offenders ($r = .36$). Psychiatrist 3 was relatively consistent (between .24 and .32) across all categories of offense and diagnosis. Finally, Psychiatrist 4 was the best able to predict psychotics ($r = .31$) and those charged with a violent offense ($r = .19$); his ratings of patients with "other" diagnosis correlated at a level of $-.33$ with DOS. These findings support the contention that, not only are some clinicians better predictors than others, but individual psychiatrists work best with certain classifications of patients.

The final problem to be addressed here concerns the elusive nature of criteria for accuracy. Given the illusory standards for "hits" and "false positives" for predictions based in a political context (Petrunik, 1983; Thornberry & Jacoby, 1979; Warren, 1979), determinants for predictive success are often rendered arbitrary, ephemeral, and meaningless (Boyd, 1980; Ennis & Litwack, 1974). In addition, earlier studies seldom employed *direct* predictions of dangerousness (but see Cooke, 1979). Nor did they in general address the notion that dangerousness outcome, like all psychosocial variables, is *continuous* rather than discrete. Not all predictions are correct or erroneous; subjects occupying middle ranges of violence and criminality on follow-up should be categorized as neither "successes" nor "failures" for the purposes of establishing accuracy. As Shapiro (1977) suggests, valid indices of predictive powers can be established only by building ranges of accuracy and failure into the appraisal.

We decided, therefore, to exclude from the determination of "hits" and "misses" all subjects who fell in the middle ranges of DOS outcome (scores from 4 to 6). Those rated at 3 or less were considered nondangerous; those at 7 or greater were positive cases. Clinicians' predictions were dichotomized; ratings of 1 (no) and 2 (low) suggested predictions of nondangerousness; 3 (medium) and 4 (high) were operationalized as positive forecasts. Table 8.7 adopts these criteria to establish, for each professional group, the relative proportions of false positives, low hits, false negatives, and high hits.

Several interesting trends emerge from these data. First, when these professionals predicted that a patient would be dangerous, they were usually wrong;

when they projected nonviolence, they were usually right. For every accurate anticipation of dangerous behavior there were for the five clinical groups the following numbers of false positives: 2.3 (psychiatrists), 3.0 (psychologists), 3.3 (social workers), 2.7 (nurses), and 2.2 (correctional officers). In contrast, the ratio of correct to erroneous predictions of nondangerousness ranged from 5.7:1 in the case of psychiatrists to 3.3:1 for social workers. An alternative measure of clinical accuracy is yielded by a comparison of false negatives and high hits; that is, of all individuals exhibiting dangerous behavior during the 24-month follow-up, how many had been predicted to be potentially violent? On these criteria, clinicians fared somewhat better, although it may be argued that this constitutes a spurious by-product of overprediction (Monahan & Cummings, 1975; Rubin, 1972; Shah, 1978; Steadman, 1976). Between 1.5 (social workers) and 3 (psychologists and correctional officers) dangerous individuals had been correctly identified for every one who was misclassified.

Overall, differential predictive skills among clinical groups appear to be more contingent on correct forecasting of nondangerous patients than on sifting out the truly dangerous. The higher prediction–outcome associations for psychiatrists (see Table 8.6) relative to other professionals are principally a function of their superior ability to detect the nonviolent. Social workers and correctional officers, in comparison, were relatively less able to classify correctly the future nondangerous clientele. Figure 8.2 compares prediction–outcome correlations for psychiatrists (best predictors) and social workers (worst predictors) by the use of a numeric scatter plot. The entire plot can be read as a visual equivalent of the Pearson product–moment correlations obtained in Table 8.6. The distribution of cases for psychiatrists represents a .20 correlation; for social workers, the association is essentially null ($r = .03$). The remarkable feature of this plot is the highly discrepant pattern of extreme scores for the two professions. For example, when psychiatrists rated a patient as not at all dangerous, 31 subjects scored 1 to 3 on outcome (only 6 patients in this range of follow-up dangerousness were so rated by social workers). Similarly, ratings of high dangerousness yielded 20 nondangerous outcomes for psychiatrists and 28 for social workers; in contrast, the social workers actually identified more 7 to 9 outcome patients as highly dangerous than did psychiatrists (12 to 9).

We conclude this section by presenting case histories of four patients: one true negative, one false negative, one true positive, and one false positive. These sketches are reconstructed from the medical records of patients, the psychiatrists' letters to judges, the brief assessment research instruments, the court disposition, and the 24-month follow-up summary. The cases were selected to illustrate several features common to success and failure in the "attribution of dangerousness" (Levinson & York, 1974). In addition, the summaries illuminate the presentation and perception of dangerous insignia during the assessment (Pfohl, 1978) and the communication of these clinical perceptions to the criminal courts.

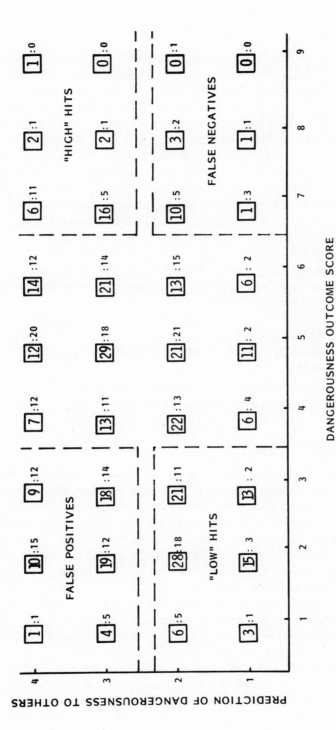

Figure 8.2. Scatter plot comparing prediction–outcome correlations for psychiatrists and social workers. Numbers in squares are psychiatrists' predictions; other numbers, social workers' predictions.

CASE 005: TRUE NEGATIVE

This individual was remanded to the BAU on a charge of being unlawfully in a dwelling house. He was a 42-year-old man with a long history
of chronic alcoholism. There was no evidence of violence in the patient's record. On examination, the accused admitted to consuming a
bottle of wine per day. The psychiatrist detected mild brain damage,
which was probably secondary to alcohol abuse. The patient was found
fit to stand trial and was not considered to be suffering from a certifiable
mental illness. It was recommended to the judge that he would be more
likely to benefit from a correctional setting than from psychiatric hospitalization. In his letter to the judge, the psychiatrist made the following observations: "Although [   ]'s life-style and individual philosophy
may reflect chronic alcohol abuse, he does not recognize any need for
further assessment or treatment. . . . [   ] showed no evidence that would
suggest he is dangerous to himself or others at the present time."

The patient was found to be of no danger to others by the psychiatrist,
psychologist, social worker, and correctional officer; the nurse was unclear on this issue. The subject was convicted on the charge and sentenced to 4 days in jail.

During the 24-month follow-up, one incident was recorded against
the subject:

A. *Criminal charges:* theft under $200 (three counts).

This received a dangerousness rating of 1.67 from the three judges.

CASE 238: FALSE NEGATIVE

This 17-year-old single man was interviewed in the BAU during the
month of May. He was originally arrested on a charge of break and
enter. During the examination he was perceived to be well oriented,
demonstrating good social judgment and "some insight into his past
difficulties handling his temper." There was no evidence of either disorder in mood or any major mental illness. The patient had spent 2½
years in a juvenile institution; for the 2 years before the current charges
he had been living on his own. The patient was working regularly in a
warehouse at the time of arrest. The psychiatrist, on this information,
recommended probation. In his letter to the judge, he wrote: "There is
no indication that [   ] represents any significant danger to the community at this time or that he is in need of any formal psychiatric treatment.
[   ] shows evidence of certain adolescent conflicts appropriate to his
age level. In the event his probation officer became concerned about

these difficulties, a psychiatric referral at that time would be appropriate.''

All five members of the interviewing team indicated that the patient was in the low range of dangerousness to others in the future. He was placed on probation for 24 months. The 24 month follow-up record reads thus:

A. *Reason for contact with hospital:* involved in violent episodes, beat up girlfriend and his best friend, frequently involved in physical fights, punched man at a dance and was prepared to strike him with a martial arts instrument, had taken a knife to a disco.

This follow-up received a rating of 7.67 from the external judges.

CASE 590: TRUE POSITIVE

This 25-year-old man was examined in December, having been remanded by the court on charges of (a) wounding and (b) weapons dangerous. The patient demonstrated a history of behavioral and emotional disorder dating back to childhood. During the interview, the accused was cooperative but displayed high levels of anxiety. In addition, he indicated excessive consumption of alcohol and methamphetamines. The examining psychiatrist found the individual fit to stand trial and free of serious mental disorder. Although he was not considered in need of psychiatric hospitalization, the patient was diagnosed to be suffering from an unspecified personality disorder with antisocial, unstable, and explosive features, further complicated by chronic alcoholism. In his letter to the presiding judge, the psychiatrist wrote: ''[   ] is a volatile youth who does pose some danger in the community, especially when drunk. This issue was discussed with him at some length and it would seem clear that he is not motivated at this stage to change his drinking patterns. Hence I believe the prognosis to be quite poor.''

All four members of the assessment team found the patient to be highly dangerous in the future. He was sentenced to 3 months in provincial prison. During the 2 years following assessment, the subject was involved in the following incidents:

A. *Criminal charges:* trafficking in narcotics, assault causing bodily harm.

B. *Misconducts during incarceration:* wilfully disobeyed a lawful order of an officer; committed or threatened to commit an assault upon another person.

C. *Reasons for contact with hospital:* hearing voices say terrible things about him and his family; overdosed on drugs; attempted suicide, mumbling to himself; threatened younger brother with an axe following an overdose of drugs while drinking beer; hearing voices talk to him about snakes and committing suicide; inappropriate giggling and smiling; smashed up mother's apartment and attempted to strangle her with a cord; alcohol abuse.

D. *Behavior during contact with hospital:* gross thought disorder; sarcastic, secretive; preoccupied with voices.

These incidents were assigned a dangerousness score of 8.67 by the independent judges.

CASE 467: FALSE POSITIVE

This patient was a 48-year-old man who was charged with (a) assault bodily harm and (b) weapons dangerous. Although he had given consent to assessment by the clinical team, he displayed evasiveness during the course of the interview. As a result, few background data were collected from the patient. The psychiatrist commented that there was "possible reluctance to cooperate in any real sense," noting that "he gave replies to questions which were at marked variance from information we possessed." The clinicians detected evidence of formal thought disorder characterized by inappropriateness, flatness of affect, and concreteness. Psychological testing supported these observations. The psychiatrist wrote the following to the presiding judge: "There would seem to be a total lack of insight by [   ] into his mental state and it was our impression that he constitutes a significant danger in the community." He recommended a 30-day assessment in a security hospital, commenting that "any further examinations of this man should only be conducted under the conditions of maximum security."

All four psychiatric team members concluded that the patient was highly dangerous to others in the future. Charges were withdrawn, and the patient was certified and detained in a security hospital for 2 years, before being transferred to a general psychiatric institution. The 2-year outcome record reads as follows:

A. *Behavior during contact with hospital:* jumping up and down on one spot and pulling his stomach in and out.

This was awarded a dangerousness score of 1.67 by the judges.

Discussion and conclusion

It is unlikely that predictions of dangerousness will recede from the medicolegal system in the near future. Considerations about future violence are reflected in discretionary decisions at every stage in the processing of deviants (Shah, 1978). As Wiggins (1973) observes, "Decisions must be made, and society must somehow go on in the absence of final solutions to the problems posed by ultimate criteria" (p. 39). Given the continued employment of forensic clinicians in the imputations of potential violence, research efforts must be directed toward a delineation of conditions under which predictions attain acceptable levels of accuracy. Empirical work based on appropriate conceptual and methodological foundations has the potential to resolve these issues.

It is important to underscore the fact that dangerousness is a legal rather than psychiatric phenomenon (Dinitz & Conrad, 1978). Clinicians who assess violence are acting within judicial and penal models and structures. This is unfamiliar terrain for medical thinking; "law presumes men to be rational, hedonistic, responsible; clinical thought provides for the probability that they may often be irrational, destructive, and most irresponsible" (Dinitz & Conrad, 1978, p. 119). At the same time, psychiatry cannot continue to perform this role in the absence of evidence demonstrating its legitimate contribution to the legal process. We argued earlier that the overwhelming proportion of literature denying the efficacy of psychiatric predictions is severely flawed by methodological deficiencies. Nevertheless, the onus is emphatically on practitioners and researchers to demonstrate this capacity. In the absence of ethical, theoretical, and empirical support, psychiatry may indeed be performing a spurious and arbitrary social control function (Petrunik, 1983; Pfohl, 1978, 1979; Steadman, 1973). Even if support is forthcoming from the social science literature, clinicians must temper their legal work with a sensitivity to the human problems issuing from predictions of dangerousness.

The current prominence of dangerousness in criminology and psychiatry is a reflection of more general concerns about the articulation between law and medicine. Those individuals who are defined as dangerous – and forensic patients more generally – are suspended between two parallel institutions that operate under vastly different ideologies and designs. Similarly, the forensic psychiatrist is saddled with competing mandates from the clinic and courtroom. As Rollin (1969) writes:

There must be far more communication between jurists and psychiatrists so that the strong arm of the law knows what the weak hand of psychiatry is doing, and even more important, perhaps, capable of doing. . . . Unless and until something of this sort is brought about, the Gilbertian situation which now obtains will continue, and psychiatrists and jurists, instead of being . . . brothers-in-law, will become increasingly partners-in-crime (p. 23).

This study represented a modest attempt to gauge the ability of clinicians to discharge one such function – the prediction, during pretrial assessment, of dangerous behavior. Although the research demonstrated moderate correlations between prediction and outcome, such assessments are severely limited by the context of the evaluation, the cross-sectional nature of the pretrial remand, the absence of critieria for operationalizing dangerousness, the failure of courts to provide feedback to the clinics, and the inattention to contextual and situational determinants of dangerous behavior. Only one clinician, a social worker who rated 16 patients, broke the .40 prediction "sound barrier." Conversely, the data indicated that clinicians vary broadly in their ability to anticipate violence and that some classes of patients may be more predictable than others. Furthermore, the evidence suggests that the major source of predictive inaccuracy resides in the failure to identify nondangerous people, that is, the relatively low proportion of true negatives. Clinicians may be advised to invert the focus of their decisions and to concentrate henceforth on the prediction of nondangerousness.

One final conclusion merits attention. In his monograph on the subject, Monahan (1981) wrote that "the inclusion of situational variables is the most pressing current need in the field of violence prediction. The principal factor inhibiting the development of situational predictors of violence is the lack of comprehensive ecological theories relating to the occurrence of violence behavior" (p. 91). It is in this area that criminology can best contribute to the forensic psychiatric process. The abundant research available in the field of criminogenesis (the study of the psychosocial and contextual determinants of criminality) should become an important resource for psychiatrists facing these kinds of prognostications. It is unlikely that predictive accuracy can be substantially advanced by this practice alone. But as any horticulturist knows, in the long term, such cross-fertilization may indeed purify the produce.

Notes

1 For a reproduction of this instrument, see Webster et al. (1982, Appendix A).
2 That is, no attempt was made at this stage to differentiate levels of dangerousness inherent in the incidents.
3 In fact, this figure underrepresents slightly the proportion of contacts. Some cases in which the nature of the contact was cursory and trivial (e.g., a drop-in), with only negligible and irrelevant information in the clinical files were excluded.
4 This operation may bias the prediction – outcome association in unknown ways. The major difficulty involves the artificial elevation of base-rate dangerousness due to the discarding of nondangerous cases. Three possible models may be in operation, all related to the interaction between level of dangerousness and magnitude of the "dark figure" (i.e., undetected dangerousness). See illustration on facing page.
   In Model 1, those individuals officially perceived to be dangerous are in fact responsible for the majority of undetected violence. The 190 subjects with no outcome records are generally nonviolent. Positive correlations between prediction and outcome are underestimates. In model 2, the absolute dark figure of dangerousness is equivalent across all levels of outcome violence, including discarded cases. Positive correlations between prediction and follow-up are unaffected by the elimination of cases with no mental health or criminal justice contacts. Although all groups are in reality more dangerous than indicated by official records, there is no interaction between level and

MODEL 1

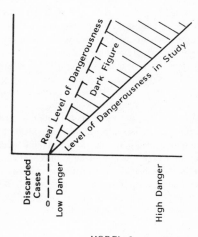

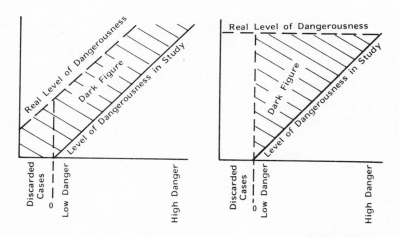

the error term. Model 3 proposes that high findings of dangerousness are spurious. Cases with low ratings, including the discarded cases, are in the aggregate equivalent in dangerousness to those with serious official records. Positive prediction–outcome correlations would be vast overestimates; a more radical version of this model would attribute even higher real levels of dangerousness to cases with low official ratings.

Theoretically, Model 2 best supports the logic followed in the present study. Because a single score of, say, 0 would be insensitive to the differences among the 190 discarded patients, their elimination would increase the power of the research. At the same time, correlations between prediction and outcome would be unchanged. The design is acceptable under Model 1, although the error term is magnified by the exclusion of the "no records" cases. Of course, the research is invalid to the degree that Model 3 reflects reality. The invalidity increases with the proportion of "low dangerous" cases detected.

5 Raters were given the following instructions: "By 'behaviours' we mean not only those in the motor–physical category (e.g., walking, grabbing), but also verbalizations (e.g., threats, yelling) and expressed thoughts or feelings (e.g., he wanted to hit someone). . . . Your task is to indicate how *dangerous* you think each follow-up profile is with respect to people other than the patient himself. You do this by circling a number from 1 to 11 for each follow-up which shows how dangerous each follow-up profile seems to *you*. You should read each of the profiles listed in the booklet and circle the number you think best fits it. If you think it is in the 'not dangerous' category, circle 1. If you think it is in the 'medium dangerous' category, circle 6. If you think it is in the 'most dangerous' category, circle 11. . . . Each of the eleven categories is an equal step on the scale of dangerousness so that '6' is one step more dangerous than '5', and '10' is one step more dangerous than '9', and so forth. . . . We would like to emphasize that your task is to choose a value which represents the degree of dangerousness inherent in *what* the individual did during two years. You are *not* to rate the individual himself and how dangerous you think he is or will be, but only the behaviours he has expressed. You will find that the majority of behaviours involve conduct directed toward other people, but if the individual acted against himself in any way, we included these behaviours as well. You are evaluating dangerousness to others only, however."

6 Pearson correlations among the three judges were .74 (Judges 1 and 2), .67 (Judges 1 and 3), and .58 (Judges 2 and 3). Distributions of their outcome ratings are indicated in the following tabulation:

	N	Mean	Median	Lowest	Highest	Standard deviation
Judge 1	404	5.24	5.69	1	11	2.30
Judge 2	406	3.54	3.15	1	9	2.04
Judge 3	407	3.78	3.58	1	9	1.75

7 For seven patients, the ratings of only two of three judges were recorded. These were averaged in the same manner as in the other cases.

8 Two variables, drug use and family social circumstances, were deleted because of large proportions of missing data.

References

Bassuk, E., & Gerson, S. Deinstitutionalization and mental health services. *Scientific American*, 1978, *238*, 46–53.

Bem, D. J., & Allen, A. On predicting some of the people some of the time: The search for cross-structural consistencies in behaviors. *Psychological Review*, 1974, *81*, 506–20.

Bem, D. J., & Funder, D. C. On predicting more of the people more of the time: Assessing the personality of situations. *Psychological Review*, 1978, *85*, 485–501.

Bottoms, A. E. Reflections on the renaissance of dangerousness. *Howard Journal.*, 1977, *16*, 70–96.

Boyd, N. Ontario's treatment of the "criminally insane" and the "potentially dangerous": The questionable wisdom of procedural reform. *Canadian Journal of Criminology*, 1980, *14*, 151–67.

Brown, H. I. *Perception, theory and commitment*. Chicago: University of Chicago Press, 1977.

Butler, B. T., & Turner, R. E. The ethics of pre-arraignment psychiatric examination: One Canadian viewpoint. *Bulletin of the American Academy of Psychiatry and the Law*, 1978, *6*, 398–404.

Cooke, G. *Follow-up of mental status of competency hearing persons.* Paper presented at the Annual Meeting of the American Psychological Association, New York, September 1–5, 1979.

Cunningham, F. *Objectivity in social science.* Toronto: University of Toronto Press, 1973.

Dershowitz, A. M. The psychiatrist's power in civil commitment: A knife that cuts both ways. *Psychology Today,* February 1969, pp. 43–7.

Diamond, B. L. The psychiatric prediction of dangerousness. *University of Pennsylvania Law Review,* 1974, *123,* 439–52.

Dinitz, S. & Conrad, J. P. Thinking about dangerous offenders. *Criminal Justice Abstracts,* March 1978, pp. 99–131.

Dix, G. E. Determining the continued dangerousness of psychologically abnormal sex offenders. *Journal of Psychiatry and Law,* 1975, *3,* 327–44.

Ennis, B. J., & Litwack, T. R. Psychiatry and the presumption of expertise: Flipping coins in the courtroom. *California Law Review,* 1974, *62,* 693–752.

Floud, J., & Young, W. *Dangerousness and criminal justice.* Totowa, N.J.: Barnes & Noble Books, 1982.

Gibbens, T. C. N., Soothill, K. L., & Pope, P. J. *Medical remands in the criminal court.* New York: Oxford University Press, 1977.

Giovannoni, J. M., & Gurel, L. Socially disruptive behavior of ex-mental patients. *Archives of General Psychiatry,* 1967, *17,* 146–53.

Gottfredson, D. Assessment of methods. In L. Radzinowicz & M. E. Wolfgang (Eds.), *Crime and justice,* (Vol. 3). New York: Basic Books, 1971.

Greenland, C., & Rosenblatt, E. M. Remands for psychiatric examinations in Ontario, 1969–1970. *Canadian Psychiatric Association Journal,* 1972, *17,* 307–401.

Gunn, J., Robertson, G., Dell S., & Way, C. K. *Psychiatric aspects of imprisonment.* New York: Academic Press, 1978.

Guze, S. B., Woodruff, R. A., & Clayton, P. J. Psychiatric disorders and criminality. *Journal of the American Medical Association,* 1974, *227,* 641–2.

Hall, H. V. Dangerousness predictions and the maligned forensic professional: Suggestions for detecting distortion of true basal violence. *Criminal Justice and Behavior,* 1982, *9,* 3–12.

Hamilton, J. R., & Freeman, H. (Eds.). *Dangerousness: Psychiatric assessment and management.* Oxford: Alden, 1982.

Henderson, S. A. From clinic to courtroom: An analysis of the content of psychiatric letters to the court. Unpublished M. A. Dissertation, University of Toronto, Centre of Criminology, 1980.

Hiday, V. A. Court discretion: Application of the dangerousness standard in civil commitment. *Law and Human Behavior,* 1981, *5,* 275–89.

Hiday, V. A., & Markell, S. J. Components of dangerousness: Legal standards in civil commitment. *International Journal of Law and Psychiatry,* 1980, *3,* 405–19.

Hinton, J. W. *Dangerousness: Problems of assessment and prediction.* London: Allen & Unwin, 1983.

Hodges, E. F. Crime prevention by the Indeterminate Sentence Law. *American Journal of Psychiatry,* 1971, *128,* 71–5.

Holland, T. R. Diagnostic labeling: Individual differences in the behavior of clinicians conducting presentence evaluations. *Criminal Justice and Behavior,* 1979, *6,* 187–208.

Klein, J. F. The dangerousness of dangerous offender legislation: Forensic folklore revisited. *Canadian Journal of Criminology and Corrections,* 1976, *11,* 109–22.

Kozol, H., Boucher, R. J., & Garafalo, R. F. The diagnosis and treatment of dangerousness. *Crime and Delinquency,* 1972, *18,* 371–92.

Laczko, A. L., James, J. F, & Alltop, L. B. A study of four hundred and thirty-five court-referred cases. *Journal of Forensic Sciences,* 1970, *15,* 311–23.

Levinson, R. M., & Ramsay, G. Dangerousness, stress, and mental health evaluations. *Journal of Health and Social Behavior,* 1979, *20,* 178–87.

Levinson, R. M., & York, M. Z. The attribution of 'dangerousness' in mental health evaluations. *Journal of Health and Social Behavior*, 1974, *15*, 328–35.

Lipton, D., Martinson, R., & Wilks, J. *The effectiveness of correctional treatment*. New York: Praeger, 1975.

Mannheim, H. *Pioneers in criminology*. Montclair, N.J.: Patterson Smith, 1960.

McGarry, A. L., et al. *Competency to stand trial and mental illness*. Washington, D.C.: U.S. Government Printing Office, 1973.

Megargee, E. M. The prediction of violence with psychological tests. In C. Spielberger (Ed.), *Current topics in clinical and community psychology*. New York: Academic Press, 1970.

Megargee, E. M. The prediction of dangerous behavior. *Criminal Justice and Behavior*, 1976, *3*, 3–21.

Mesnikoff, A. M., & Lauterbach, C. G. The association of violent dangerous behavior with psychiatric disorders: A review of the recent literature. *Journal of Psychiatry and Law*, 1975, *3*, 415–45.

Mischel, W. *Personality and assessment*. New York: Wiley, 1968.

Monahan, J. *The clinical prediction of violent behavior*. Rockville, Md.: National Institute of Mental Health, 1981.

Monahan, J. & Cummings, L. Social policy implications of the inability to predict violence. *Journal of Social Issues*, 1975, *31*, 153–64.

Morris, N. *The future of imprisonment*. Chicago: University of Chicago Press, 1974.

Petrunik, M. The politics of dangerousness. *International Journal of Law and Psychiatry*, 1983, *5*, 225–53.

Pfeiffer, E., Eisenstein, R. B., & Dabbs, E. G. Mental competency evaluations for the federal courts. 1. Methods and results. *Journal of Nervous and Mental Disease*, 1967, *144*, 320–28.

Pfohl, S. J. *Predicting dangerousness: The social construction of psychiatric reality*. Lexington, Mass.: Heath, 1978.

Pfohl, S. J. From whom will we be protected? Comparative approaches to the assessment of dangerousness. *International Journal of Law and Psychiatry*, 1979, *2*, 55–78.

Price, R. R. Psychiatry, criminal law reform and the 'mythophilic' impulse: On Canadian proposals for the control of the dangerous offender. *Ottawa Law Review*, 1970, *4*, 1–61.

Quinsey, V. L. The baserate problem and the prediction of dangerousness: A reappraisal. *Journal of Psychiatry and Law*, Fall 1980, pp. 329–40.

Quinsey, V. L., Warneford, A., Preusse, M., & Link, N. Released Oak Ridge patients: A follow-up study of review board discharges. *British Journal of Criminology*, 1975, *15*, 264–70.

Rappeport, J. R. *The clinical evaluation of the dangerousness of the mentally ill*. Springfield, Ill.: Thomas, 1967.

Rennie, Y. F. *The search for criminal man: A conceptual history of the dangerous offender*. Lexington, Mass.: Heath, 1978.

Ribner, S. A., & Steadman, H. J. Recidivism among offenders and ex-mental patients. *Criminology*, 1981, *19*, 411–20.

Roesch, R., & Golding, S. L. *Competency to stand trial*. Champaign–Urbana: University of Illinois Press, 1980.

Rollin, H. R. *The mentally abnormal offender and the law: An inquiry into the working of the relevant parts of the Mental Health Act, 1959*. Oxford: Pergamon, 1969.

Rothman, D. J. *Conscience and convenience*. Boston: Little Brown, 1980.

Rubin, B. Prediction of dangerousness in mentally ill criminals. *Archives of General Psychiatry*, 1972, *27*, 397–408.

Sarbin, T. The dangerous individual: An outcome of social identity transformations. *British Journal of Criminology*, 1967, *7*, 285–95.

Sasowsky, L. Crime and violence among mental patients reconsidered in view of the new legal relationship between the state and the mentally ill. *American Journal of Psychiatry*, 1978, *135*, 33–42.

Sawyer, J. Measurement and prediction, clinical and statistical. *Psychological Bulletin*, 1966, *66*, 178–200.

Schreiber, A. M. Indeterminate therapeutic incarceration of dangerous criminals: Perspectives and problems. *Virginia Law Review*, 1970, *56*, 602–34.

Scott, P. Assessing dangerousness in criminals. *British Journal of Psychiatry*, 1977, *131*, 127–42.

Scull, A. T. *Decarceration: Community treatment and the deviant – A radical view*. Englewood Cliffs, N.J.: Prentice-Hall, 1977.

Segal, S. P., & Aviram, U. *The mentally ill in community-based sheltered care: A study of community care and social integration*. New York: Wiley, 1978.

Shah, S. A. Dangerousness and civil commitment of the mentally ill: Some public policy considerations. *American Journal of Psychiatry*, 1975, *132*, 501–5.

Shah, S. A. Dangerousness: A paradigm for exploring some issues in law and psychology. *American Psychologist*, 1978, *33*, 224–38.

Shapiro, A. R. Evaluation of clinical predictions. *New England Journal of Medicine*, 1977, *296*, 1509–14.

Steadman, H. J. The psychiatrist as a conservative agent of social control. *Social Problems*, 1973, *20*, 263–71.

Steadman, H. J. Predicting dangerousness. In D. J. Madden & J. R. Lion (Eds.), *Rage, hate, assault and other forms of violence*. New York: Spectrum, 1976.

Steadman, H. J., & Cocozza, J. J. *Careers of the criminally insane*. Lexington, Mass.: Heath, 1974.

Steadman, H. J., & Cocozza, J. J. Psychiatry, dangerousness and the repetitively violent offender. *Journal of Criminal Law and Criminology*, 1978, *69*, 226–31.

Steadman, H. J., & Morrissey, J. P. The statistical prediction of violent behavior: Measuring the costs of a public protectionist versus a civil libertarian model. *Law and Human Behavior*, 1981, *5*, 263–74.

Taylor, I., Walton, P., & Young, J. *The new criminology: For a social theory of deviance*. London: Routledge & Kegan Paul, 1973.

Thornberry, T. P., & Jacoby, J. E. *The criminally insane: A follow-up of mentally ill offenders*. Chicago: University of Chicago Press, 1979.

Van Dine, S., Conrad, J. P., & Dinitz, S. *Restraining the wicked: The incapacitation of the dangerous criminal*. Lexington, Mass.: Heath, 1975.

Vold, G. *Theoretical criminology*. New York: Oxford University Press, 1958.

von Hirsch, A. *Doing justice: The choice of punishments*. New York: Hill & Wang, 1976.

Waller, I. *Men released from prison*. Toronto: University of Toronto Press, 1974.

Warren, C. A. B. The social construction of dangerousness. *Urban Life*, 1979, *8*, 359–84.

Webster, C. D., Menzies, R. J., & Jackson, M. A. *Clinical assessment before trial*. Toronto: Butterworths, 1982.

Wenk, E., Robison, J. & Smith, G. Can violence be predicted? *Crime and Delinquency*, 1978, *18*, 79–84.

Wiggins, J. S. *Personality and prediction: Principles of personality assessment*. Reading, Mass.: Addison-Wesley, 1973.

Wolfgang, M. An overview of research into violent behavior. Testimony before the U.S. House of Representatives Committee on Science and Technology, 1978.

Zitrin, A., Hardesty, A., Burdock, E., & Drosaman, J. Crime and violence among mental patients. *American Journal of Psychiatry*, 1976, *133*, 142–49.

9 Prediction at the system level: measuring the presumed changes in the clientele of the criminal justice and mental health systems

Henry J. Steadman

In chapter 8, Menzies, Webster, and Sepejak describe an attempt to predict the likelihood that individual mentally disordered offenders will behave violently in the future. It is, in fact, the case that the previous chapters have been concerned with issues related to the individual: the procedural problems involved in identifying who will be violent, the implications of making those predictions, the results of making certain types of errors in those predictions, the development of technologies for the identification of individuals who may be violent, and in some instances the whole vexing matter of public policy considerations in making such predictions. The essential point is that in every instance my fellow authors have dwelled on the individual.

This emphasis on the individual is the antithesis of the discussion in this chapter. I have tried to capture this in the title of the piece. I want to look at the facilities that are involved in the systems of care for people who are thought to be violent, people who are involved in both the criminal justice and the mental health systems. I wish to discuss how these systems may be changing. My idea is to focus not on the individual client, but on the *flow* of clients. Are the characteristics of these client groups changing? If they are changing, there will be implications for the way in which the systems are structured. The task of clinicians and the public policy implications of the prediction of violent behavior may be very much different depending on how the systems are working and how they are interacting with one another. We think that our data, although based on recent research in the United States, will have relevance to Anglo-American

This chapter is a product of a large-scale study, "The Movement of Offender Populations Between Mental Health and Correctional Facilities," funded in part by the National Institute of Justice (79-NI-AX-0126). John Monahan was the coprincipal investigator who contributed equally to any success of this endeavor. Eliot Hartstone, Barbara Warner Duffee, and Pamela Clark Robbins all made essential contributions through their dedicated work of data collection and analysis.

145

practices in general. The specific issues and the era in which the issues have developed may be different, but the general policy questions about who is responsible for what types of people under what types of circumstances do seem to be generally similar across settings.

The title of this chapter may seem unwieldly. The word "prediction," although chosen to fit the general theme of this volume, is not entirely apt. It is intriguing that, when we want to talk about changes at the system level, we do not use words and concepts like "prediction" and "prognosis" (as in chapter 4). Instead, we tend to talk about "forecasts" and "projections." We use a different language – the language of the urban planner, the program planner. We talk about long-range planning.

Playing out these semantic differences, we examined the dictionary to see if our intuitive reaction was accurate. On the basis of *Webster's Collegiate Dictionary,* we would suggest that, in fact, these terms could almost be used interchangeably. "Forecasting" is defined as "calculating or predicting, usually as a result of rational study and the analysis of pertinent data." In effect, we are forecasting dangerousness or forecasting violence, but we use the term "prediction." In terms of projections, there are people at the provincial or state level who do projections all day on incomes, economic status, size of prison populations, and so on. The dictionary defines what they are doing as "estimating the future possibilities, based on current trends." That is really what we are doing with the individual when we are predicting dangerousness. We are estimating the future probabilities. Yet when we talk on the system level, we use a different language, and it is this that accounts for the present, slightly unusual and awkward title. Nevertheless, when we say that we are "projecting" what the prison population will be or "forecasting" what the mental health population will comprise, we are making predictions. We are making predictions about facilities, institutions, and systems rather than individuals. So although the language is different, the basic problem is still the same – making accurate forecasts.

Specific issues

The specific issues with which I deal here can be seen from a number of perspectives. The first vantage point is that of the federal government bureaucrat, not using that term in a pejorative sense. The others are those of the correctional administrator, the mental health clinician or practitioner, and the academic. In my view, the set of issues has been framed quite differently by each of those groups. In the United States, one federal perspective is that forecasters have been particularly poor at making accurate projections of the size of prison populations. As Stone stated in chapter 1, the prison population in the United States has gone up dramatically in the past 5 years. The prisons are simply bulging. Legislators are now pressing to pass prison-construction bond issues. A major problem has been that when people projected prison population size for the 1980s in the early 1970s they were markedly wrong. Some federal agencies have recently started to ask, "Why did we make such poor predictions? We knew what the demographics were; we knew what the birth rate of the population was; we knew about the aging-in process in the population. We had some sense of what crime rate trends tend to be. Why did we make such poor predictions?" One of the possible answers is that these agencies did not take enough consideration of what was happening in the mental health system (Law Enforcement Assistance Administration, 1979). To understand what was going to happen in the prison system, it may also have been necessary to look at what was going to happen in the mental health system. The expansion and contraction of the clientele in the mental health system may, in fact, have had a very direct impact on the prison system.

From the correctional administrators' standpoint, it is impossible to go to a sheriffs' or administrators' conference anywhere in North America, whether for correctional staff, front-line workers, or senior officials, and not hear the refrain: "My facility cannot operate properly because I have all these disturbed people who ought to be in the mental health system. Why do I have these people? They don't belong in prison. They don't belong in corrections." In the United States such statements are very pervasive. There is a strong belief that, in the 10-year period of deinstitutionalization of the mental health system, a large number of "crazies" ended up in the prison system, and this impeded correctional programs. These, we are told, are the people who cause trouble. Although there have been numerous organized prison riots for racial and economic purposes, the aspect of prison life considered to create the most trouble for front-line correctional officers or correctional administrators is the number of mentally deranged people populating the prisons and jails (Bonovitz & Bonovitz, 1981; Reveron, 1982; Wilson, 1980).

The staff in the state mental hospitals, however, have their own "tune to sing." There, the front-line staff, whether they are in charge of admissions, acute-care, or long-term units (but particularly admissions and acute-care services), consistently complain that their clientele are more difficult than they ever have been before. They contend that, compared with the patients they treated in the 1960s and early 1970s, these patients are younger, tend more often to be male, and tend to be much more aggressive and assaultive. The staff's interpretation of the situation is that the criminal justice system personnel do not want to deal with these people, and they are dumping young, violent, black, intractable men in the state hospitals. In some instances these individuals are deposited by criminal orders and some cases by involuntary civil commitment under the dangerousness aegis (Abramson, 1972; Geller & Lister, 1978; Lamb & Grant, 1982).

Thus, there seem to be very contrasting points of view. On the one hand, mental health staff at the state hospitals are claiming that all of these people belong in a correctional system. On the other, the correctional staff are asserting that all of these "crazies," who by rights should be in mental hospitals, are being very disruptive and ruining the correctional rehabilitation program.

Finally, we come to the fourth vantage point, that of academics. We use this term to include people who write in professional journals. In these periodicals, there is consistent mention of the criminalization of mentally disordered behavior (Abramson, 1972; Rachlin, Pam, & Milton, 1975). The idea here is that with the deinstitutionalization movement has come an increase in the number of disturbed and disturbing people in the community (Sosowsky, 1978; Whitmer, 1980; Zitrin et al., 1976). This, it is explained, is the result of the closing down of state hospitals. This heightened level of disruptive behavior required some type of societal response. The academics argue that the reason there were more disturbed people in the community was that the mental health system had basically closed up shop. Not only had the mental health system decreased the number of available beds, but it had also set more restrictive hospital admission standards. Deinstitutionalization involves closing the front door by setting up new admission standards, conducting more effective screening, and simply not letting people in. These people may be geriatric patients who belong in a nursing home because they have physical rather than mental ills or people who are, on the face of it, able to function with some type of community support system (often enthusiastically but loosely defined and frequently more inadequate than would have been thought possible). As a result of fewer beds and more restrictive admission standards, so the argument goes, arrest was the available alternative for coping with the high levels of disturbed behavior in the community. Society had no option but to book individuals of this type into some sort of custodial situation. They had to be taken off the street and, perhaps in some instances, funneled into the mental health system by means of one criminal procedure or another. They could not be admitted via civil commitment.

These, then, are the federal, correctional, mental health, and academic perspectives. There are some points of agreement. Academics seem to be supporting correctional administrators by saying that the correctional system has been radically changed by the state mental hospital deinstitutionalization. Mental health staff recognize that their system has, indeed, changed and think that they, too, have the wrong clientele in their system.

Who is right? Did mental health advocacy, mental health attorneys, and changing commitment codes really produce these effects? Have the responsibilities of the two systems really changed? Is it possible that both sides are right? Is it an either/or question? These are the questions we had in mind when we began the research project described in the following section. During the 1970s had the clientele of the one system actually changed in relation to the other? Although there had been much talk about these issues, no one had any data. To our knowledge, there is not one published article in the North American literature comparing data obtained before with data collected after deinstitutionalization and examining the clientele of those two systems before and after. We therefore held no brief for either side.

Current research

The study reported here focused on two time points, the years 1968 and 1978. These years were selected because, as should be clear, they suited our purposes quite well and also because of certain practicalities. We wanted to choose a time when deinstitutionalization had not yet been fully implemented. The problem is that deinstitutionalization is not a unidimensional concept. It happened in different ways, at different places, at different times (Morrissey, 1982). It is not a standard phenomenon at all, although it is often talked about as if it were. The year 1968 can perhaps be established as a point when the state of California was farthest along and the state of New York was entering into the process of deinstitutionalization very vigorously. Most other states were not far underway. The main practical reason for selecting 1968 was that we doubted if we could find data for earlier years. This, after all, is a limiting consideration. It is wonderful to come up with elaborate research designs and multiple data points, but if one does not have hard data, it is not possible even to approach the main questions of interest. The second data point was, as noted, 1978. The study was started late in that year so that the available information would be the most recent. These two years gave us a 10-year period in which to look at the changes that may have occurred.

We concentrated on the "confinement careers" of the population, an inappropriate term as it happens. We were interested in the basic question, Had the clientele of the two systems changed over that 10-year period? Because we could not examine all aspects of the issue, we decided to focus on the questions in terms of arrest, incarceration, and mental hospitalization histories. These taken together we called confinement careers. Arrest really is not confinement, which is why the concept is slightly inapt. Six states were selected for study. Our choice of states was determined partly by happenstance and partly by the fact that we had access to the necessary data. Readers of this book will recognize that obtaining access to medical and correctional files is seldom easy; state-level records are difficult to come by.[1] So we selected states where we had contact people in the key state agencies who would have the data we needed. In negotiating these arrangements we aimed to achieve a geographic range of states. The states that we selected were California, Arizona, Texas, Iowa, New York, and Massachusetts. Despite the fact that, to some extent we had to take what we could get, the states studied are reasonably representative of the United States as a whole. Thus, we can draw some generalizations about the country as a whole from these six states.

We selected a random sample of all admissions in 1968 and 1978 to the state prison system, and we took a random sample of all mental patients who came into the state hospital system in those two years. As well, we drew a random sample of "quasi offenders" (defendants incompetent to stand trial, individuals not guilty by reason of insanity, mentally disordered sex offenders, which only two of the six states had, and transfers from prison to mental hospitals, i.e., convicted persons serving time who were considered to be in need of care and transferred to a mental health setting). The third group is not dealt with here. Across the six states we had a sample of 3,896 inmates, 2,376 patients (and 1,452 quasi offenders). Our interest was this: Did inmates and state hospital patients appear to be different in 1978 from those in 1968 in regard to their arrest records, incarceration records, and mental hospitalization records?

Findings

Table 9.1 presents data on the proportion of patients who came into the mental health system with prior arrest records. The question here is, Are more prisoners coming into the correctional system with hospitalization histories, or are more mental patients being admitted to mental health institutions with arrest records? To put it differently, are some of the clientele from the mental health system now shifting into the correctional system, or are criminal justice clientele shifting into the mental health system?

Table 9.1 shows that in five of the six states, Iowa being the exception, the proportion of patients with prior arrests *increased* over the 10 years. With the six states combined in 1968, 38% of all male patients (admissions) had prior arrest records as compared with 56% in 1978. Interestingly, we found that the mental patients admitted in 1978 also had a higher proportion of prior mental hospitalizations (45% versus 54%). In all six states the number with prior hospitalizations had increased. This is interesting given the conceptualization that, with fewer beds and more restrictive mental health commitment codes, fewer people were being admitted to state hospitals. In fact, the number of *episodes* of care in the U.S. state mental hospital system changed relatively little between 1955 and 1975 (Morrissey, 1982). The number of patients residing in the facilities decreased dramatically, but the average length of stay also decreased dramatically. The number of admissions remained almost constant. The number of episodes of care given in a state mental hospital system changed relatively little during the era of deinstitutionalization. The present data are consistent with this

Table 9.1. *Percentage of mental hospital admissions with prior arrests, 1968 and 1978*

State	1968	1978
New York	36.7	51.0
California	32.8	65.3
Arizona	32.6	47.5
Texas	37.0	49.0
Iowa	55.6	42.9
Massachusetts	56.0	62.6
Mean (weighted)	38.2	55.6

in that the proportion of inpatient admissions with a prior hospitalization went from 45% in 1968 to 54% in 1978.

Table 9.2 compares prisoners in 1968 with those in 1978. This is the counterpart of Table 9.1. That is, How many prisoners coming into the system had hospitalization histories? The findings here are very inconsistent. In three of the states the proportion went up, and in three of the states it went down. Overall, it changed relatively little. In 1968 an average of 8% of prisoners came into the system with prior hospitalization. In 1978 it increased to about 11%, overall. Texas contributed most of that. There is little support in these two tables for the correctional perspective as articulated earlier. However, the data also suggest that this cross-sectional view may be somewhat misleading. The reader will recall that, among the mental patients as a group, there was not only a higher proportion with arrests, but also a higher proportion with mental hospitalizations. That is, they were coming into both systems more often. The revolving-door idea seems to include not only the revolving hospital door, but also the revolving cell door.

To explore these issues further, we examined the career patterns of these study groups. We identified four major patterns: (a) all individuals coming into either system for the first time, that is, first arrest or first mental hospitalization; (b) individuals with only prior hospitalizations; (c) individuals with only prior criminal justice contact, that is, arrest or incarceration; and (d) individuals with both prior mental health and criminal justice experiences. More prisoners coming in with only mental health histories would suggest that a new correctional clientele were coming from the mental health system. In other words, if people who had, for example, four prior mental hospitalizations had started entering the prison system for the first time in 1978, that would suggest a possible transfer of responsibility. Reciprocally, a greater proportion of 1978 mental patient admissions with multiple prior arrests but no prior hospitalizations would suggest a

Table 9.2. *Percentage of prison admissions with*
prior state mental hospitalizations, 1968 and 1978

State	1968	1978
New York	12.1	9.3
California	9.5	15.2
Arizona	3.9	2.2
Texas	0.3	8.4
Iowa	7.7	16.7
Massachusetts	12.5	9.0
Mean (weighted)	7.9	10.4

shift in the responsibility from the criminal justice to the mental health system. Less clear are the issues involving people who have bounced back and forth between the two systems, often for many years. Our feeling was that if, in the case of the people who had both mental health and criminal justice histories, the first "event" was some mental health problem, especially if they had experienced a whole series of mental health events before any criminal justice events, that would suggest some shift of disturbed people from the mental health to criminal justice system. Reciprocally, if someone coming into the mental health system in 1978 had numerous prior criminal justice events and had hospitalizations only late in his or her "confinement career," that would suggest a shift of responsibility from the mental health to criminal justice system.

As Table 9.3 shows, in terms of prisoners, almost nothing changed between 1968 and 1978. Just as with the cross-sectional approach that demonstrated little overall change in the proportion of prisoners with hospitalizations in 1978, little changed with regard to career patterns. There were only relatively minor changes across the six states. It turns out, not surprisingly, that prisoners in both years had almost no mental health events at all. The proportion with any prior mental health events at any time in their careers (Patterns 2 and 4) ranged from only 2% (Arizona) to 17% (Iowa). In 1968, it was even lower, ranging from .3% in Texas to 12% in New York and Massachusetts. This group of people coming into the state prison system had clearly not bounced back and forth between the mental health and criminal justice systems. This group clearly had not been entirely in the mental health system for years and finally, after deinstitutionalization, in prisons as institutions of last resort. The prisoners' histories in both years almost exclusively involved criminal justice.

In contrast, the mental patients changed greatly, particularly in terms of the percentage of those coming into the system with no prior events (Pattern 1). As is evident in Table 9.4, the trend is consistent across all six states. The number of patients with no prior system contacts diminished in all six states. In contrast,

Table 9.3. *Patterns in the confinement careers of prison admissions, 1968 and 1978*

State	Pattern 1: No prior CJ or MH events		Pattern 2: Prior MH event(s) only		Pattern 3: Prior CJ event(s) only		Pattern 4: Prior MH and CJ events	
	1968 (%)	1978 (%)	1968 (%)	1978 (%)	1968 (%)	1978 (%)	1968 (%)	1978 (%)
New York	7.9	3.8	0.5	0.0	79.9	87.0	11.7	9.3
California	1.5	3.5	0.0	0.0	89.0	81.3	9.5	15.3
Arizona	8.4	11.4	0.0	0.0	87.7	86.4	3.9	2.3
Texas	14.4	13.0	0.0	0.3	85.3	78.6	0.3	8.0
Iowa	15.6	17.4	1.0	1.0	76.5	65.9	6.9	15.7
Massachusetts	11.0	10.8	0.0	0.0	76.6	80.1	12.5	9.0
Mean (weighted)	9.2	9.3	0.3	0.2	80.2	80.2	7.7	10.3
	(N = 179)	(N = 179)	(N = 5)	(N = 4)	(N = 1,606)	(N = 1,550)	(N = 150)	(N = 199)

Note: CJ and MH denote criminal justice and mental health, respectively.

Table 9.4. *Patterns in the confinement careers of state mental patient admissions, 1968 and 1978*

State	Pattern 1: No prior CJ or MH events		Pattern 2: Prior MH event(s) only		Pattern 3: Prior CJ event(s) only		Pattern 4: Prior MH and CJ events	
	1968 (%)	1978 (%)	1968 (%)	1978 (%)	1968 (%)	1978 (%)	1968 (%)	1978 (%)
New York	30.9	24.0	32.4	25.0	13.9	15.9	22.8	35.1
California	38.2	21.9	29.0	12.5	17.8	28.3	15.0	37.2
Arizona	46.9	33.3	19.8	19.2	21.9	26.3	11.5	21.2
Texas	44.0	28.6	19.0	22.4	20.0	20.4	17.0	28.6
Iowa	28.3	26.5	16.2	20.6	29.3	15.3	26.3	27.6
Massachusetts	31.9	19.8	12.1	17.6	33.0	24.2	23.1	38.5
Mean (weighted)	35.6	24.4	26.1	20.0	19.2	21.9	19.1	33.7
	(N = 418)	(N = 286)	(N = 307)	(N = 235)	(N = 225)	(N = 257)	(N = 224)	(N = 396)

those with prior contacts with both systems (Pattern 4) increased in all six states. This was true for those coming into the system with both types of events whether they started with the criminal justice event or a mental health event. There were increases from 1968 to 1978 in five of six states for both types of career pattern.

We would summarize these data as follows. There was almost no change in the proportion of prisoners with prior state mental hospital experiences. There is no indication that the number of prisoners in the state prison system with mental health problems, as shown by history of hospitalization, changed. However, there was consistent change in the characteristics of the mental patients coming into the state system. They were much more active, particularly with more arrests. They had also had more hospitalizations.

The next question that has been articulated in the literature on the effects of deinstitutionalization is whether patients coming into the mental health system have more arrests because it is only by laying charges that the police can remove them from the street (Abramson, 1972; Lamb & Grant, 1982). If they are acting in a bizarre fashion or if they are disturbing people, the mental hospital will not necessarily take them. In 49 of the United States' 50 jurisdictions, ''dangerousness'' is the major requirement for involuntary civil commitment. Someone who is simply acting up, bothersome, or even bizarre does not necessarily meet that standard. Arguably, then, the police must charge such people with a low-grade misdemeanor, harassment, disorderly conduct, or something similar. If this is a typical pattern, our data would show that a disproportionate number of mental patients were being arrested for nuisance types of offenses. We would see not only that a higher proportion were being arrested, but also that the type of offenses were changing.

If, however, the mental health perspective is more accurate, that is, mental health staff have to deal with more violent, aggressive, hostile people, then the arrests that were accumulated during this period would be more violent in nature. In 1968 of all the arrests accumulated by the people coming into the mental health systems, 12% were violent (i.e., murder, attempted murder, assault and battery, violent sex offenses, and kidnapping). About 63% were nuisance type of offenses. In the 1978 group the proportion of arrests that were violent increased to 20%. The percentage of offenses that were of the nuisance type decreased from 63% of the arrests to 38%. There was also a substantial increase in drug and property offenses.

Our interpretation at this point is that all three of the indicators we have studied suggest that there has been a definite shift from the criminal justice to mental health system, whereas the latter has remained very stable. The proportion of mental patients with prior arrests nearly doubled across the six states over the 10-year period. The proportion of offenders with any prior state mental hospital contacts was quite constant. Finally, the offense distribution of patient arrests reflects slightly more violent and property offenses and considerably fewer nuisance types of offense. There is no support for the corrections perspective that the clientele of that system are more deranged than they were 10 years ago, before the mental hospitals were deinstitutionalized.

Discussion

It seems from our data that what has changed most about criminal justice's mental health problems are the perceptions of correctional administrators. This was vividly brought home when we were making a site visit at a county jail in California. We asked its administrator if the kind of people (in regard to mental health issues) in his jail were any different from those a decade earlier. He said, "No! Ten years ago when these people gave us trouble, we threw them in the tank for a week. Now we send them to mental health." At one time, the inmate who threw his feces, who attacked other inmates, who screamed and kept the cell block awake all night simply was considered a "pain in the ass." He was thrown in the hole. Now, he is sick; the correctional administrator calls the psychologist and says, "Get this guy down to the mental health unit and get him on some meds. He's driving everybody crazy. He doesn't belong in this unit." The behavior of the inmate has not changed. The perception of what is wrong and the expectation of who should respond to it have changed. It is not the sergeant on the unit who will react by transporting the inmate to the hole. It is the psychologist in the psychiatric unit who is now expected to respond.

What we hear and see in corrections today may be a prime example of mental health salesmanship. Correctional administrators have been convinced that mental health can "keep the lid on" their facilities. They really do not care about traditional mental health treatment. However, they have been convinced that bringing in mental health practitioners will help to keep some equilibrium in their jails and prisons. In fact, they are probably right. Where they have developed mental health units or where they have had the ability to transfer patients out of the correctional facility to a mental health unit, their life has been much easier. Things have settled down, and in many instances inmates have actually improved. The disruptive behavior seems to have declined – at least until the inmates who have been transferred to mental health units come back to the jail or prison, and then it starts all over again. They then wonder why the mental health personnel have sent them back to the jail and cannot see that they are still sick.

As a result of this, correctional staff see many "crazies" among the inmates in their jails and prisons. They claim that they were not there 10 years ago. They were. The staff just looked at them differently; they responded to them differently. We find no support for the perception that the changes in the mental health system at the state prison level caused any measurable changes in the clientele in the state prison system.

I would like to point out now that there is a major flaw in the argument I have been developing. The data presented here deal with *state* mental hospitals and *state* prisons. I would argue that the major impact of deinstitutionalization, if there has been one, is at the local level, that is, at the local lockup, where the arrestee is kept for 24 or 48 hours until arraignment or bail or until transfer to the county jail, and at the county jail. At the state prison level, the clientele are of a different type. They have long records; very rarely are they there on first offenses.

If the mental health system has stopped admitting some types of people and shifted that responsibility to the correctional system, the probable impact would be at the local level. That is where the screening for the whole state or provincial system occurs. If the police cannot deliver someone to the emergency room of the general hospital or to the admitting unit at the provincial or state mental hospital, what are they going to do with him? In fact, they have to book him. When they book him, they bring him to the local lockup or the county jail, and that is where he stays, depending on the speed with which he is processed, for a substantial period of time. If there is going to be a problem, a suicide attempt particularly, that is where it is going to happen. Nevertheless, in terms of volume of admissions and seriousness and acuteness of problems, the local jail is a much more important mental health arena than the provincial, state, or federal prison system.

From a research standpoint, these retrospective studies are extremely difficult to conduct. It is not easy to reconstruct data of this kind. Unless somewhere there are much better data systems than we have seen, the cost of reconstruction is very nearly prohibitive. What we really need are prospective studies. The only way to acquire the kind of information actually needed is to start now and see what happens. When we try to reconstruct, we end up with many gaps. It is not possible to be nearly as definitive (not that most research is extremely definitive anyway), but at least there is a better chance of an unambiguous outcome if a prospective rather than a retrospective model is being used.

Finally, I would like to make a few points about the use of prediction. Up to this point we have dealt with prediction at the system level: projecting or fore-casting the shape of custody systems in corrections and mental health. I would suggest that the issue of the prediction of dangerousness of the individual will never go away. A cursory examination of the history of mental health institutions in the public sector shows that this issue has always existed. Society can be told this or that, but in the end it has always demanded that someone, usually the physician, make predictions, and on the basis of those estimates someone is preventatively detained on grounds of being mentally ill. Such mechanisms will, I suspect, always be with us in some form.

There is some possibility, however, that if the criminal justice system were used more often as an alternative to the civil mental health system, the issue of the prediction of dangerousness would diminish dramatically. To admit people into mental health treatment because they are in need of treatment *after* they have been arrested requires no demonstration of dangerousness. There is no medical estimation of future probabilities of dangerousness. Once a person deemed in need of treatment is in the correctional criminal justice system, before trial or after conviction, he or she can usually be transferred. According to a U.S. Supreme Court decision, *Viteck v. Jones,* an inmate in the United States has a right to a hearing before the transfer can occur. But the hearing is related only to the issue of need of treatment. It is a medical question. It is not the legal question of dangerousness. It is irrelevant once the person has been sidetracked via the criminal justice system. So to the extent that the criminal justice system assumes a dominant role in delivering clients to the mental health system, I propose that the issue of the prediction of individual dangerousness becomes much less important.

Nonetheless, the probability that predictions will remain a core public policy issue for psychiatry is high. The probability that forecasts and projections of the needs of the mental health and criminal justice systems will systematically take into consideration each other's projections is low, although these predictions at the system level are as crucial as most of those at the individual level. The circumstances in which clients find themselves may be very much dependent on those predictions, forecasts, and projections at the system level. These estimates deserve substantially more attention both from planners, who use the language of forecast and projection, and from clinicians, who speak the language of prediction and prognosis, because institutional practice situations ultimately are structured by system-level changes.

Notes

1 A more detailed study would take into account the number of mentally disordered persons incarcerated in local jails and lockups. It is just possible that the characteristics of such a sample might differ from our state-level groups and that a study conducted over time, as in the present venture, might reveal differences.

References

Abramson, M. The criminalization of mentally disordered behavior: Possible side effect of a new mental health law. *Hospital and Community Psychiatry,* 1972, *23,* 101–5.
Bonovitz, J., & Bonovitz, J. Diversion of the mentally ill into the criminal justice system: The police intervention perspective. *American Journal of Psychiatry,* 1981, *138,* 973–76.

Geller, J., & Lister, E. The process of criminal commitment for pretrial psychiatric examination: An evaluation. *American Journal of Psychiatry,* 1978, *135,* 53–60.

Lamb, R., & Grant, R. The mentally ill in an urban county jail. *Archives of General Psychiatry,* 1982, *39,* 17–22.

Law Enforcement Assistance Administration. *The movement of offender populations between mental health and correctional facilities.* Washington, D.C.: U.S. Government Printing Office, 1979.

Morrisey, J. P. Deinstitutionalizing the mentally ill: Process, outcomes and new directions. In W. R. Grove (Ed.), *Deviance and Mental Illness.* Beverly Hills, California: Sage, 1980.

Rachlin, S., Pam, A., & Milton, J. Civil liberties versus involuntary hospitalization. *American Journal of Psychiatry,* 1975, *132,* 189–91.

Reveron, D. Mentally ill and behind bars. *American Psychological Association Monitor,* March 1982.

Sosowsky, L. Crime and violence among mental patients reconsidered in view of the new legal relationship between the state and the mentally ill. *American Journal of Psychiatry,* 1978, *135,* 33–42.

Whitmer, G. From hospitals to jails: The fate of California's deinstitutionalized mentally ill. *American Journal of Orthopsychiatry,* 1980, *50,* 65–70.

Wilson, R. Who will care for the mad and the bad? *Corrections Magazine,* 1980, *6,* 23–31.

Zitrin, A., Hardesty, A. S., Burdock, E. I., & Drosaman, J. Crime and violence among mental patients. *American Journal of Psychiatry,* 1976, *133,* 142–9.

10 Criteria for civil commitment: medicolegal impasse

Barry A. Martin

Historical context

Throughout recorded history societies faced with the enigmatic, sometimes frightening behavior of the mentally ill have attempted to formulate suitable explanations and solutions consonant with both the prevailing scientific "truths" and the *Zeitgeist*. Those believed to be demoniacally possessed were exorcised or executed. Later, more enlightened explanations led to more "therapeutic" solutions such as extended voyages on "ships of fools," an early variant of the socially acceptable policy of keeping the insane out of sight.

The late eighteenth and nineteenth centuries witnessed the emergence of the belief in environmental causes of insanity. Consistent with this belief, the mainstay of treatment was considered to be refuge from the noxious influences of the environment. Asylums were built and "moral therapy" was employed to counter the psychological stresses thought to be causal. The results were considered so gratifying that the demand, stimulated by reformist zeal, soon swamped the facilities. Asylum and moral therapy gave way to custodialism (Sederer, 1977).

The period from the 1850s to the 1940s was the snake pit era of mental hospitals. Staffing and financing were inadequate to provide moral treatment. In the absence of both knowledge of the causes of insanity and effective treatments, the socially acceptable solution was simply reversion to keeping the insane out of sight. During this period it was relatively easy for people to put away intolerable individuals. This was partially offset by crusades for commitment laws to prevent wrongful incarceration. These formed the basis for current legislation on involuntary hospitalization (Slovenko & Luby, 1975).

The 1940s ushered in the era of community psychiatry. Coupled with the advent of the psychopharmaceutical treatment revolution and the philosophy of wholesale community management of mental disorders spawned by that revolution, the observation of certain detrimental effects of institutionalization was followed by the quantum, and fallacious, leap in logic to the conclusion that any hospitalization was potentially harmful and to be avoided or minimized. Suddenly, institutions were considered causal and the solution was to reintroduce patients to the environment that was formerly considered causal. A considerable literature documents the consequences of this social policy (Arnhoff, 1975; Bachrach, 1976; Becker & Schulberg, 1976; Kirk & Therrien, 1975). It is well summarized by Arnhoff (1975):

The major public policy decisions, however, have tended to ignore substantive issues and developments in biological psychiatry and the behavioral sciences and have been predominantly determined by short-range political expediency and the pressures of social reform. A compelling body of systematic evidence now exists to suggest not only that the actual cost-benefits of community treatment (using cost in its broadest social sense) are far less than its advocates proclaim, but that the consequences of indiscriminate community treatment may often have profound iatrogenic effects; in short, we may be producing more psychological and social disturbance than we correct (p. 1277).

It is not inconceivable that the prevailing attitudes and assumptions regarding the place of hospital-based treatment of the mentally ill have come to bear on the formulation of social policy regarding involuntary hospitalization. It is within this historical context that the current issues of civil commitment legislation must be examined. This chapter addresses one aspect of such legislation, the behavioral criteria for involuntary hospitalization, with only secondary consideration of the legal procedures for the review of cases.

The Mental Health Act of Ontario and recent amendments

The passage of controversial amendments (such as Bill 19 in 1978) to the 1967 Mental Health Act of Ontario may well be illustrative of the process whereby public policy tends to be "predominantly determined by short-range political expediency and the pressures of social reform" (Arnhoff, 1975, p. 1277). Certainly the paucity of objective data marshaled in support of the amendments is as remarkable as the plethora of rhetoric (Anand, 1979; Szasz, 1978) in the debate and the literature dealing with civil commitment legislation. Before 1967, the criterion for civil commitment in Ontario was that an individual be "suffering from such a disorder of the mind that he requires care, supervision and control for his own protection or welfare, or for the protection of others" (Mental Hospitals Act of 1960). This wording, in particular the term "welfare," relied too heavily on the doctrine of *parens patriae* such that a more narrowly defined criterion was sought. Under the 1967 Mental Health Act, the ill-defined conditions that were to be present before a person could be involuntarily committed to a psychiatric facility were observable indications "that he/she suffers from a mental disorder of a nature or degree so as to require hospitalization in the interests of his/her own safety or the safety of others" and that the person "is not suitable for admission as an informal patient." An explicit intent of the amended act (1978) was to reduce the ambiguity of the term "safety" by redefining the criteria for involuntary admission as the presence of observable facts leading the physician "to believe that the person (a) has threatened or attempted or is threatening or attempting to cause bodily harm to himself; (b) has behaved or is behaving violently towards another person or has caused or is causing another person to fear bodily harm from him; or (c) has shown or is showing a lack of competence to care for himself'' and, further, that "the physician is of the opinion that the person is apparently suffering from mental disorder of a nature or quality that likely will result in (d) serious bodily harm to the person; (e) serious bodily harm to another person; or (f) imminent and serious physical impairment of the person.'' Thus, the concept of "safety" has been narrowly restricted to that of physical integrity.

The logic of this amendment would be apparent if the usual reason for involuntary hospitalization were to prevent individuals from physically injuring themselves or others. There is, however, some evidence that the vast majority of patients who are involuntarily hospitalized are so managed for reasons other than the prevention of physical injury. The principal civil libertarian position is that there is no other justification for involuntary hospitalization. It would appear that the implicit intent of this amendment to the act is in accord with the civil libertarian argument. Interpreted literally, it would preclude the hospitalization of many of those so managed in the past. A frequently stated assumption is that the intent of the 1967 act was to restrict the grounds for commitment to that of physical danger, and therefore the amendment simply introduces a precision of language rather than a narrowing of the criteria. A more cautious assumption would be that the wording of the act was deliberately left open to a wider interpretation in recognition of the fact that there were a number of circumstances that might require involuntary admission in the absence of more satisfactory feasible alternatives. Parenthetically, it also seems inappropriate to dismiss completely the notion of psychological harm to the self or others when considering the potential consequences of mental disorders. Such a separation of physical from psychological harm is reminiscent of Cartesian mind–body dualism.

Proponents of the amendments have argued that many patients involuntarily hospitalized could be managed with greater recourse to "community and family support and resources" (Timbrell, 1978). Although laudable in intent and consistent with the tenets of community psychiatry, the belief in the presence of satisfactory feasible alternatives "in that nebulous but benign fastness called the community" (Kedward, 1975, p. 3) fails to take cognizance of the fact that certain fundamental premises of the community psychiatry approach to the management of mental disorders may be more apparent than real. A considerable literature (Arnhoff, 1975; Bachrach, 1976; Becker & Schulberg, 1976; Kirk & Therrien, 1975) has demonstrated that a great deal of time is required to develop community agencies that can adequately coordinate their services to replace those provided by the hospitals. Other considerations that tend to undermine assumptions about the proposed alternatives are that many of those with severe mental disorders are often unable to avail themselves of community-based services and, further, that by the time a person has reached the point where involuntary hospitalization is even being considered, the available family supports have often been completely exhausted.

In view of the importance of this issue, there has been a relative scarcity of thorough investigations of the circumstances under which people have been admitted involuntarily and the process whereby such important decisions have been made in order to ascertain the necessity, or lack of necessity, for recourse to commitment and to document the frequency of any abuse of the intent of the Mental Health Act. The failure to put reliable numbers to the unavoidable instances of incorrect application of any legislation, no matter how carefully worded, precludes an accurate interpretation of the overall significance of those instances (i.e., are they isolated examples or evidence of systematic abuse of the intent of the legislation?).

During the course of an earlier study of trends of admission to psychiatric facilities (Martin, Kedward, & Eastwood, 1976), some of the data were suggestive of a certain consistency over time in the use of involuntary commitment. Although there has been a dramatic increase in the total rate of admission in the past few decades, expressed as a rate per unit of population, admissions for the severe mental disorders (psychoses) have remained relatively constant over time. This is consistent with the fact that there is no compelling evidence that the incidence of psychotic disorders has changed significantly in several decades. Expressed as a rate per unit of population, the use of the involuntary certificate for admission has tended to correlate with the steady rate of admission for severe disorders rather than with the dramatically increasing total rate of admission for all disorders. Thus, it seems to have been used with some degree of consistency over a period. This is suggestive of use based on clinical judgment that has been quite consistent over time rather than misuse based on fluctuating, idiosyncratic interpretation. The relatively constant rate (relative to the total admission rate) of use of the involuntary certificate reflects the fact that there continues to be a fairly constant incidence and prevalence of severe mental disorder considered in need of treatment and, failing treatment, temporary protection or asylum. Despite the purported ambiguity of the 1967 act, this fairly consistent interpretation over decades during which there have been major changes in treatment philosophy suggests a certain validity to the clinical criteria for commitment. The clinical decision-making process would appear to be independent of legislation and, if so, it is expected that recent amendments to the act will not appreciably affect the rate of involuntary hospitalization.

Civil libertarian position

A quotation from Mill's "On Liberty" is frequently cited by civil libertarians in opposition to involuntary commitment. Indeed, the quotation was used by the

Ontario minister of health in an address to the legislature in support of amendments to the Mental Health Act of Ontario (Timbrell, 1978): ''The only purpose for which power can be rightfully exercised over any member of a civilized community, against his will, is to prevent harm to others. His own good, either physical or moral, is not sufficient warrant. He cannot rightfully be compelled to do or forbear because it will be better for him to do so, because it will make him happier, because, in the opinions of others, to do so would be wise, or even right.'' Not only is this quotation most often used completely out of context, but it indicates an extremely superficial interpretation of Mill's thinking. In the present context it also fails to take cognizance of Mill's upbringing under the Benthamite philosophy that took no account of the emotional and often irrational basis of human behavior. The next paragraph of the essay considers those incapable of mature reason to be exempt from his doctrinaire statement (see Monahan, 1977). However, legal reformists and commitment abolitionists also reject the doctrine of *parens patriae,* which permits the imposition of treatment for a person's own good.

The dilemma that precludes the reconciliation of a strict civil libertarian view and the practice of commitment is that timeworn question of whether there is such a thing as mental illness (Moore, 1975). Unfortunately, either one accepts that there are severe mental disorders, an integral part of which is impaired judgment as to the presence of illness, the need for treatment, and the likelihood of favorable response to treatment, or one does not accept such entities. If the existence of such severe mental disorders is accepted, then there is usually little difficulty in acknowledging the argument that civil libertarian positions are certainly the ideal for rational people but that the principles ring hollow when one is attempting to deal with irrational behavior and its consequences. A refusal to accept the existence of such disorders leads to an inability to accept that the unique circumstances may require some compromise of the ideal.

Legal versus medical concepts

As noted, one of the stated objections to the wording of the 1967 Mental Health Act lay in the vague definition of the criteria for commitment. This vagueness is anathema to legal thinking in the criminal justice system, which quite rightly demands a very stringent definition of conduct sufficient to warrant a loss of freedom. Of necessity, legal definitions must reject vague and controversial psychiatric definitions of sickness in favor of more easily described aspects of behavior. In this regard, the paper ''On Being Sane in Insane Places'' (Rosenhan, 1973) has had undue influence in view of the substantive criticism of its scientific merit (Spitzer, 1976). Nevertheless, the notion of ostensibly normal people being misdiagnosed as psychotic and admitted to a mental hospital is sufficiently disquieting as to discredit in the minds of many the psychiatric definition of mental illness. The reported adulteration of the nosology (Reich, 1975) to serve political ends furthers the public perception of psychiatric diagnosis as a very fallible exercise. In order to offset this fallibility it has been considered appropriate to draw analogies between the process of civil commitment of the mentally ill and the due process of the criminal justice system.

With respect to the criteria for civil commitment, legal due process is concerned with both the definition of behavior sufficient to warrant a loss of liberty and the evidentiary standards of proof that such a definition is met in any given case. Of course, the two concepts must go hand in hand. The most precise definition is of little use if there are no valid, or at least reliable, means of determining the degree of concordance between the facts of a case and the definition. Unfortunately, the amended criteria for commitment seem to have been drafted with insufficient attention to this point. Restriction of the concept of ''safety'' to that of physical integrity is an attempt to gain a precision of definition more consonant with the principles of legal due process. Because the infliction of physical injury per se either is subject to no sanctions or is the subject of criminal law and the sanctions of the court, such behavior requires the presence of mental disorder to bring it within the terms of reference of civil commitment legislation. Although one might reasonably argue that a certain precision is possible in the description of behavior deemed physically injurious or even threatening of physical injury, that precision is lost when combined with the description of behavior deemed to indicate the presence of mental disorder that is likely to result in physical harm or injury. With respect to clarity of definition, the weak link remains the definition of mental disorder and the inherent components of severe mental disorder that made it the subject of commitment legislation in the first instance. Part of that weakness is due to a great ignorance of the significance of much behavior that occurs in the context of mental disorder such that the prediction of physical harm is often no better than chance. Furthermore, unlike the criminal justice system dealing with events that have occurred in the past, the civil commitment process is often used as a remedy for anticipated behavior. Thus, with respect to the issue of physical danger, despite homage to due process principles by those who would amend the legislation, the civil commitment process is actually an instrument for preventive detention. This mutual incompatibility suggests that there is a clear limitation to the extent to which one may apply legal concepts of due process to civil commitment. Alternatively, zealous advocates of the application of due process might interpret this sort of incompatibility as a clear indication of a need to abolish civil commitment.

With respect to the evidentiary standards of proof that a given case meets the criteria for civil commitment, one is faced with an even greater discrepancy between the law and the state of the art of psychiatry. In civil law the standard is that of a preponderance of the evidence, whereas criminal law requires proof beyond a reasonable doubt. A decision by the U. S. Supreme Court (*Addington v. State of Texas*, 99 Supreme Court 1804, 1979) set an intermediate standard for commitment: "clear and convincing" evidence that the person is both mentally ill and dangerous. It is useful to examine this American judgment because U.S. jurisprudence has had an inordinate influence on Canadian legislation.

In his review of the standard of proof concept, Chief Justice Burger noted the underlying principles of distributing the risk of error in judgment, in this context between society and the patient, and of weighing the relative importance of the outcome of litigation. In rejecting the civil standard, Burger concluded that, because a possible outcome of commitment litigation involves a loss of liberty, an element shared with criminal cases, the distribution of the risk of error should decidedly favor the individual over society such that a mere preponderance of the evidence is insufficient to justify commitment. The criminal standard attempts to minimize the risk of error to the individual at the risk to society of allowing some who are guilty to go free. In rejecting this standard, Burger writes:

It may be true that an erroneous commitment is sometimes as undesirable as an erroneous conviction . . . it is not true that the release of a genuinely mentally ill person is no worse for the individual than the failure to convict the guilty. One who is suffering from a debilitating mental illness and in need of treatment is neither wholly at liberty nor free of stigma. . . . It cannot be said, therefore, that it is much better for a mentally ill person to "go free" than for a mentally normal person to be committed (*Addington v. State of Texas*, p. 1810).

Burger goes on in his judgment to note the fallibility of psychiatric diagnosis and the impossibility of meeting the criminal standard, noting that the state is not required to guarantee error-free convictions or to adopt standards of proof that "may completely undercut its efforts to further the legitimate interests of both the state and the patients that are served by civil commitments" (*Addington v. State of Texas*, p. 1806).

Unfortunately, with respect to both the diagnosis of mental disorder and the prediction of dangerousness psychiatrists are hard pressed to meet even the civil standard of proof, let alone the aforementioned intermediate standard. Once again, this aspect of due process appears to be meaningless when applied to civil commitment. Despite the spurious impression of a greater correctness in the application of civil commitment measures as a result of grafting the due process of the criminal justice system to the civil commitment procedure of the mental health system, the fundamental differences in the problem at issue must lead to a failure of the graft. The failure to recognize the limited applicability of due process in this instance is reminiscent of the failure to take cognizance of the state of the art of psychiatry in the formulation of the Durham rule and the resultant disillusionment (Bazelon, 1974).

Much of the apparently irreconcilable debate in this area stems from the differences in conceptualizing the problem by lawyers and psychiatrists. This is succinctly summarized in an article by Chodoff (1976):

The lawyers see and are concerned with the failures and abuses of the process. Furthermore, as a result of their training, they tend to apply principles to classes of people rather than to take each instance as unique. The psychiatrists, on the other hand, are required to deal practically with the singular needs of individuals. They approach the problem from a clinical rather than a deductive stance. As physicians, they want to be in a position to take care of and to help suffering people whom they regard as sick patients. They sometimes become impatient with the rules that prevent them from doing this (p. 501).

Stone (1977) has cogently presented the potential consequences of overzealous application of due process safeguards to psychiatric decision making. He appropriately rejects the implicit analogy between the mental health system and the criminal justice system and suggests that reforms premised on these analogies may adversely affect the provision of care to the mentally ill. In describing the typical response of psychiatrists to the adversary process, he states that "they are not implacable adversaries determined to retain their power over patients" (p. 276). This is certainly consistent with the observation that most clinicians would defend the premise that involuntary hospitalization is used as a last resort and only after much effort is expended to provide the least restrictive alternative management for the patient. Indeed, many clinicians find the commitment process a necessary evil and apply it only after much soul searching. The suggestion (Steingarten, 1977) that this circumspect approach is only a belated response to legal due process safeguards is invidious. Stone, a psychiatrist with a good knowledge of mental health law, summarizes his opinions as follows: "The legal solutions secured in the courtrooms have established an impressive edifice of due process, but beyond that legal structure human suffering continues unabated and its relief is more difficult to achieve. At the very least, in reviewing recent mental health litigation and its effects, the question must be asked, Is it really the patients who have had their day in court?" (p. 278).

A lead article in the *American Journal of Psychiatry* outlines a commitment law that purports to bridge the medicolegal gap. In this paper Roth (1979) appears to suggest a retention of broad criteria for commitment through the obfuscating splitting of the procedure into *parens patriae* and police power (dangerousness) types of commitments. Unfortunately, the proposed procedure for *parens patriae* commitment, modified from that of Stone (1975b), contains criteria as ambiguous and undefinable as the concepts of safety and dangerousness. Under this proposed system, the continuance of involuntary status is dependent on a demonstration of legal incompetency to consent to or refuse treatment. (Although Roth distinguishes between incompetency and the usual clinical criterion of impaired judgment, the difference is largely semantic.) However, as noted by both Roth (1979) and Steingarten (1977), there is no satisfactory test for competency in the civil commitment context. Therefore, to premise commitment criteria on a nonexistent capacity to determine competency does not appear to advance the state of the art. Steingarten's critique of Stone's proposed commitment criteria would therefore apply equally to Roth's variation on a theme. Furthermore, the criteria for assessing competency proposed by Roth for trial applications are tautologous in that the patient who *understands* the consequences of his continued behavior and the rationale for and potential benefits of the proposed treatment is not going to be subject to civil commitment in the first instance. Such a degree of understanding does not obtain concurrently with the sort of mental status that has traditionally led to commitment in Canada. In addition, the determination of such understanding is fraught with all the difficulties now present in the determination of insanity as a defense under the Canadian Criminal Code. The appreciation of the nature and quality of acts in the criminal justice system requires the same integrity of mental status as does the degree of understanding implied by the competency criteria proposed by Roth. It is quite doubtful that the measurement of this aspect of mental status can be done more reliably in the civil commitment context than is currently done in criminal cases.

With respect to the criteria for initial commitment, the *parens patriae* court hearing proposed by Roth would occur after a brief period during which the patient would already, in effect, have been committed, presumably (although this is quite unclear in Roth's article) on the grounds that "absent treatment the immediate prognosis is for major distress of the person" (Roth, 1979, p. 1122). "Major distress" does not lend itself to more precise definition than does "safety" or "dangerousness." Police power or dangerousness commitments under Roth's proposal deal only with physically violent but competent patients who may be more suitably managed in a penal rather than a therapeutic setting. Dangerousness-to-self commitments are also dependent on the likelihood of physical harm to the self as are the amended Ontario criteria. It is concluded that this proposed commitment law does not address the fundamental dilemma with respect to the actual criteria for commitment.

Issue of dangerousness

A considerable literature is devoted to improving the predictability of dangerousness and to criticizing psychiatrists for their inability to do so. However, there are very persuasive arguments that dangerousness should not be an issue with respect to involuntary hospitalization. Rather, the issue is whether mental illness has impaired the capacity to make an informed decision regarding treatment. As summarized by Peszke (1975), "To limit involuntary commitment to those who are considered dangerous is to assert that only those who are sick and dangerous can be treated, while those who are sick but not dangerous would be abandoned. Committing a mentally ill individual to a hospital because he or she fulfills the criteria of dangerousness while not committing a nondangerous mentally ill person who is incapable of making rational decisions and could benefit from treatment is analogous to not hospitalizing an unconscious accident victim who is unable to ask for help but is not dangerous'' (p. 827).

Stone (1975b) has placed the notion of dangerousness in proper perspective as a criterion for civil commitment:

It is surprising how long the notion of a unitary, calculable quantity known as dangerousness has persisted, both in statutes and judicial decisions. Only rarely have courts asked the component questions of the magnitude, likelihood, preventability, and likely victims of the alleged dangerous conduct. Furthermore, surrounding the process of civil commitment of dangerous persons is the profound question of why only the allegedly mentally ill should be subject to this form of preventive confinement – especially since the evidence suggests that of all the candidate variables, mental illness is an especially poor indicator of future criminal conduct. One court has said that without ''an analytical framework to guide . . . courts in applying the conclusory term 'dangerous to others' . . . [it] . . . could readily become a term of art describing anyone who we would, all things considered, prefer not to encounter on the streets.'' And the current system seems to confirm this concern. But a careful definition of dangerousness as the sole standard to be proven by a preponderance of the evidence will solve none of the important problems, except in the sense that it would put an end to involuntary commitment (p. 49).

At this point the unfortunate lack of association between dangerousness and *treatable* mental disorder should be emphasized. Although there appears to be some association of violent acts with mental illness (Rubin, 1972), the association may largely be with specific diagnostic groups, particularly the personality disorders. It should be noted that there is no uniform agreement among psychiatrists that people with personality disorders are mentally ill, although they may well be dangerous. Even if considered to be mentally ill, those individuals with character disorders who commit violent acts are often difficult or impossible to treat. In such cases the notion of treatability becomes central if the institution of choice for that person is to be a hospital. Logically, the absence of illness and of treatment should preclude hospitalization. One might argue that the purely asylum function of a mental hospital constitutes treatment for those in crisis in order to justify commital. After crisis resolution, for those who are untreatable the hospital environment is inappropriate. As Stone (1975a) says, ''If commitment is not based on treatability but on dangerousness, emergency commitment becomes almost nothing but preventive detention, which has, of course, been anathema to civil libertarians on a variety of constitutional grounds'' (p. 830).

With respect to the prediction of dangerousness, the statistics on the prediction of low base-rate events indicate that such prediction is not, and likely never will be, sufficiently accurate to make it an appropriate criterion for civil commitment. The ratio of false to true positives yielded by even the most accurate predictive instruments is not acceptable. Stone (1975b) uses the following illustration: "Assume that one person out of a thousand will kill. Assume also an exceptionally accurate test is created which differentiates with 95% effectiveness those who will kill from those who will not. If 100,000 were tested, out of the 100 who would kill, 95 would be isolated. Unfortunately, out of the 99,900 who would not kill, 4,955 people would also be isolated as potential killers'' (p. 27). Because the suicide rate in Canada is approximately one-seventh of that used in the example (approximately 0.13 per thousand population, Statistics Canada, 1979) the number of false positive predictions of suicide would be much higher. The predictive accuracy of current techniques is much less than 95%.

Reasons for involuntary admission

Recourse to involuntary hospitalization is a second-order decision made after the decision that the patient requires admission to hospital. A number of studies have addressed the variables influencing the decision to hospitalize a patient, and a few studies have compared groups of voluntary and involuntary patients with respect to these variables. There is little uniformity among the findings of the latter studies. In a study by Spensley et al. (1974), 79% of involuntarily admitted patients had agreed to voluntary hospitalization or had been discharged within 5 days of admission. The median length of involuntary hospitalization was 3 days. The patients were admitted to a facility oriented toward crisis intervention and outpatient therapy. In studies based at state mental hospitals, Gove and Fain (1977) found that 67% of involuntarily admitted patients were discharged within 38 days, and Zwerling et al. (1975) found that 30% were discharged in 3 months compared with 70% of voluntary patients. The latter two studies revealed that the severity of symptoms differentiated the groups, the more severe being committed. This contrasts with the findings of Dawson (1972), as discussed later. Gove and Fain noted that committed patients tended to have fewer social and economic resources than voluntary patients. The sociological study by Rushing (1971) also indicated an inverse relationship between civil commitment and socioeconomic status. These results are consistent with the epidemiology literature (Dohrenwend & Dohrenwend, 1969), which clearly documents the increased prevalence of severe mental disorder – that most likely to be managed by civil commitment – and low socioeconomic status.

A British study (Dawson, 1972) of 50 involuntarily admitted patients matched by diagnosis to a group of voluntarily admitted patients showed that only 13 (26%) patients were involuntarily admitted because of danger to themselves or others. There was no difference in the degree of disturbed behavior exhibited by the two groups. There was no significant difference in a number of demographic variables examined. Only the factor of denial of illness differentiated the groups, the involuntarily admitted demonstrating significantly more marked denial with consequent refusal to enter hospital voluntarily.

In some cases, admission was enforced in order to forestall anticipated social or family disruption or future violent behaviour. Such decisions were based on the pattern of past events. In other cases, the decision turned on the hardship and suffering caused to the patient's family which, although not amounting to physical violence, *nevertheless went far beyond the limits of what is ordinarily regarded as tolerable.* . . . However, since these reasons for admission occurred quite as often in the voluntarily admitted as in the compulsorily admitted group, they provide no explantion why an order was necessary, whether or not violence had occured or been threatened. In fact, by far the most dangerous individual in the whole group was admitted voluntarily (p. 228, emphasis added).

The results of a study (Perrin, 1973) of the information recorded on a sample of certificates for involuntary admission to an Ontario mental hospital have been used to support the argument that many people are unnecessarily committed. The slightly biased and rhetorical hypothesis of the study was as follows: "That the concept 'mental illness' is such an abstract, unreliable, meaningless term as to make it impossible to commit people on this basis, that they are instead committed for somehow annoying others, for upsetting society in some way by their presence" (p. 4). This study categorized the information contained on 200 randomly selected commitment forms and found that only 22 (11%) of the forms could be considered to contain information sufficient to fulfill the legislated criteria for commitment. The author equated "safety" with "dangerousness" and concluded that reasons other than dangerousness were responsible for most admissions. Earlier studies by Page and Yates (1973, 1974) revealed that only 22% of commitment forms made any reference to dangerousness. These authors concluded that the introduction of the 1967 Mental Health Act appeared to have little influence on physicians' practices.

It is of considerable interest that an exhaustive review of civil commitment legislation in Massachusetts (McGarry & Schwitzgebel, 1978) as well as a Canadian study (Page & Firth, 1979) did not take the methodology of investigating reasons for involuntary admission any farther than previous studies that have examined the documentation of those reasons on civil commitment forms. Comparable results were forthcoming. It may be possible to conclude from the consistency of these studies that physicians by and large have poorly documented the reasons for involuntary admission. The conclusion that involuntary admission was unnecessary cannot be drawn from this kind of study.

Conclusion

The medical profession may have too quickly acceded to societally imposed tasks of great difficulty. A case in point is the prediction of dangerousness and the application of civil commitment procedure by physicians. Nevertheless, because most civilized countries have civil commitment legislation, it would appear that someone has to perform this function. It is suggested that recent attempts to eliminate ambiguity in the civil commitment legislation in Ontario have paradoxically made this difficult task more difficult, assuming that the main objective of such legislation is to act in the best interests of those with severe mental disorders. Thus, psychiatrists literally interpreting the legislation are forced to do that which they have been proved incapable of doing in order to treat certain mentally disordered individuals. In forcing psychiatrists to base the decision for involuntary hospitalization solely on the criterion of dangerousness, one obliges them to use a criterion that would result in an excessively high number of false positive commitments. Psychiatrists are trained to diagnose and treat treatable mental disorder, which most often is not associated with physically dangerous behavior. Legislation that associates dangerous behavior with mental illness and makes such an association a prerequisite for the treatment of some of those patients with severe mental disorders simply disregards the natural history of most severe psychiatric syndromes.

Despite a well-taken concern about the inadequate documentation of the reasons for civil commitment, there has been no substantive evidence for large-scale or systematic abuse of the basic intent of civil commitment legislation in Canada. In the absence of such evidence, it is incumbent on those who would alter the legislation to demonstrate clearly that patients admitted involuntarily have been so admitted unnecessarily. It would have been preferable had such investigations been done before the introduction of recent amendments to the Mental Health Act in Ontario. Too often social policy is formulated in the absence of this necessary documentation. With respect to treatment policy for the mentally ill, this process has been described well by Arnhoff (1975):

Throughout the greater part of human history the role of the medical man in the care and treatment of the mentally ill has been a minor one. Only in recent decades has the medical approach assumed a dominant position in this field. . . . conceptions of mental illness and the treatment afforded those labelled mentally ill have reflected prevailing religious, moral and social philosophies. . . . the major trends in the field continue to be dominated by social philosophy, moral suasion, and belief under the guise of medicine (p. 1278).

Perhaps nowhere is this more apparent than in current trends in the hospitalization of the mentally ill, in particular involuntary hospitalization. Objective investigation is imperative if social policy is to be formulated on something less ephemeral than moral suasion.

The statement by Roth, Meisel, and Lidz (1977) in reference to competency is equally applicable to the criteria for commitment: ''Unless it is recognized that there is no magical definition of competency to make decisions about treatment, the search for an acceptable test will never end. 'Getting the words just right' is only part of the problem. In practice, judgements of competency go beyond semantics or straightforward applications of legal rules; such judgements reflect social considerations and societal biases as much as they reflect matters of law and medicine" (p. 283). The current medicolegal impasse with respect to the criteria for civil commitment will not be resolved unless the social considerations are more fully appreciated.

In its attempts to deal with this insoluble problem that will not go away, society has simply failed to accept that the current state of ignorance precludes a valid solution. Instead, society tends to resort to the application of an elaborate procedure on the beguiling assumption that a solution emerging from that procedure will possess a validity achieved by adherence to legal mechanisms and concepts. That spurious validity is the cul-de-sac into which the conflicting legal and medical thinking has led and out of which must come a better solution that is truly in the best interests of afflicted patients and their families.

References

Anand, R. Involuntary civil commitment in Ontario: The need to curtail the abuses of psychiatry. *Canadian Bar Review, 1979, 57,* 250–80.

Arnhoff, F. N. Social consequences of policy toward mental illness. *Science, 1975, 188,* 1277–81.

Bachrach, L. L. *Deinstitutionalization: An analytical review and sociological perspective* (National Institute of Mental Health, Department of Health, Education, and Welfare Publication No. ADM 76–351). Washington, D.C.: U. S. Government Printing Office, 1976.

Bazelon, D. L. The perils of wizardry. *American Journal of Psychiatry, 1974, 131,* 1317–22.

Becker, A., & Schulberg, H. C. Phasing out state hospitals: A psychiatric dilemma. *New England Journal of Medicine, 1976, 294,* 255–61.

Chodoff, P. The case for involuntary hospitalization of the mentally ill. *American Journal of Psychiatry, 1976, 133,* 496–501.

Dawson, H. Reasons for compulsory admission. In J. K. Wing & A. M. Hailey (Eds.), *Evaluating a community psychiatric service.* London: Nuffield Provincial Hospitals Trust, Oxford University Press, 1972.

Dohrenwend, B. P., & Dohrenwend, B. S. *Social status and psychological disorder.* New York: Wiley, 1969.

Gove, W. R., & Fain, T. A comparison of voluntary and committed psychiatric patients. *Archives of General Psychiatry, 1977, 34,* 669–76.

Kedward, H. B. Home treatment versus hospital treatment: Asylum agonistes. *Canadian Psychiatric Association Journal, 1975, 20,* 3–5.

Kirk, S. A., & Therrien, M. E. Community mental health myths and the fate of former hospitalized patients. *Psychiatry, 1975, 38,* 209–17.

Martin, B. A., Kedward, H. B., & Eastwood, M. R. Hospitalization for mental illness: Evaluation of admission trends from 1941 to 1971. *Canadian Medical Association Journal, 1976, 115,* 322–25.

McGarry, A. L., & Schwitzgebel, R. K. *Civil commitment and social policy* (Public Health Service Grant MH 25, Final Report). Cambridge, Mass.: Harvard Medical School, Laboratory of Community Psychiatry, June 30, 1978.

Monahan, J. John Stuart Mill on the liberty of the mentally ill: A historical note. *American Journal of Psychiatry, 1977, 134,* 1428–9.

Moore, M. S. Some myths about "mental illness." *Archives of General Psychiatry*, 1975, *32*, 1483–97.

Page, S., & Firth, J. Civil commitment practices in 1977: Troubled semantics and/or troubled psychiatry. *Canadian Psychiatric Association Journal*, 1979, *24*, 329–34.

Page, S., & Yates, E. Civil commitment and the danger mandate. *Canadian Psychiatric Association Journal*, 1973, *18*, 267–71.

Page, S., & Yates, E. Semantics and civil commitment. *Canadian Psychiatric Association Journal*, 1974, *19*, 413–14.

Perrin, B. T. *Involuntary commitment to mental hospitals: Why?* Unpublished Master of Arts thesis. Toronto: York University, 1973.

Peszke, M. A. Is dangerousness an issue for physicians in emergency commitment? *American Journal of Psychiatry*, 1975, *132*, 825–8.

Reich, W. The spectrum concept of schizophrenia. *Archives of General Psychiatry*, 1975, *32*, 489–98.

Rosenhan, D. L. On being sane in insane places. *Science*, 1973, *179*, 250–8.

Roth, L. H. A commitment law for patients, doctors, and lawyers. *American Journal of Psychiatry*, 1979, *136*, 1121–7.

Roth, L. H., Meisel, A., & Lidz, C. W. Tests of competency to consent to treatment. *American Journal of Psychiatry*, 1977, *134*, 279–84.

Rubin, B. Prediction of dangerousness in mentally ill criminals. *Archives of General Psychiatry*, 1972, *27*, 397–407.

Rushing, W. A. Individual resources, societal reaction, and hospital commitment. *American Journal of Sociology*, 1971, *77*, 511–26.

Sederer, L. Moral therapy and the problem of morale. *American Journal of Psychiatry*, 1977, *134*, 267–72.

Slovenko, R., & Luby, E. D. On the emancipation of mental patients. *Journal of Psychiatry and the Law*, 1975, *2*, 191–213.

Spensley, J., Barter, J. T., Werme, P. H., & Langsley, D. G. Involuntary hospitalization: What for and how long? *American Journal of Psychiatry*, 1974, *131*, 219–33.

Spitzer, R. L. More on pseudoscience in science and the case for psychiatric diagnosis. *Archives of General Psychiatry*, 1976, *33*, 459–70.

Statistics Canada. *Causes of death in 1976*. Catalogue 84-203 annual, Ottawa, 1979.

Steingarten, J. L. Book review of A. A. Stone's *Mental health and law: A system in transition. Journal of Psychiatry and the Law*, 1977, *5*, 625–37.

Stone, A. A. Comment (on Peszke, 1975). *American Journal of Psychiatry*, 1975, *132*, 829–31. (a)

Stone, A. A. *Mental health and law: A system in transition* (National Institute of Mental Health, Department of Health, Education, and Welfare Publication No. ADM 76-176). Washington, D.C.: U.S. Government Printing Office, 1975.(b)

Stone, A. A. Recent mental health litigation: A critical perspective. *American Journal of Psychiatry*, 1977, *134*, 273–9.

Szasz, T. The case against compulsory psychiatric interventions. *Lancet*, 1978, *1*, 1035–6.

Timbrell, D. Statement to the motion for second reading of Bill 19. Ontario Legislature, Toronto, April 11, 1978.

Zwerling, I., Karasu, T., Plutchik, R., & Kellerman, S. A comparison of voluntary and involuntary patients in a state hospital. *American Journal of Orthopsychiatry*, 1975, *45*, 81–7.

11   Prediction, professionalism, and public policy

Bernard M. Dickens

The medical specialty of psychiatry and its related discipline of clinical psychology have received distinguishing recognition in this century through their practitioners' involvement in the management of the violently disturbed. The mental health professions have gained charge of those who appear to pose a danger to the safety of others or to the safety of themselves. As madness became elevated from the depraved depths of sin and demonaic possession to occupy the morally neutral condition of adverse and menacing humor and then to achieve the sympathetic and protected status of illness, the prestige of professional involvement with the demented rose accordingly. Prisons for the mad became hospitals and mental health centers, their captors became physicians and therapists, and their inmates became patients (Hunter & Macalpine, 1963).

The self-confidence that developed in the mental health professions as a product of prestige and a protected field of practice withstood the studies accumulating in the professional literature from about the middle of this century that questioned and doubted the accuracy, validity, and reliability of psychiatric diagnoses (e.g., Ash, 1949) and of predictions of behavior (e.g., Glaser, 1955). After the late 1960s, critics of considerable stature presented the inaccuracies of clinical psychiatric predictions (e.g., Dershowitz, 1969), particularly of dangerousness (e.g., Diamond, 1974; Ennis & Litwack, 1974; Kozol, Boucher, & Garofalo, 1972). Practitioners continued to present expert testimony, however, in criminal trials including sentence hearings and delinquency dispositions, in dangerous offender proceedings aimed at perhaps indeterminate preventive detention,[1] at bail hearings and proceedings before parole boards, and in civil commitment proceedings resulting in involuntary detention of nonoffenders found to possess potentially harmful characteristics. Mental health professionals and organized psychiatry made little apparent response to criticisms in forensic and therapeutic practice, until the decision of a superior court in California in the 1974 case of *Tarasoff v. Regents of the University of California.*[2] An appeal of the case was entered in the Supreme Court of California, and by the time this was heard in 1976,[3] organized psychiatry had come officially to deny the possession of a professional skill to predict individual dangerousness accurately. The implications for professionalism and for public policy of this perception by psychiatry of its modest predictive skills are the subject of this chapter. Because the *Tarasoff* case was the apparent turning point, however, it may be appropriate to outline initially its material elements.

On October 27, 1969, an overseas student at the University of California killed Tatiana Tarasoff, the girl to whom he had an emotional attachment.[4] Two months earlier, the student had expressed his intention to kill her to a psychologist employed at the university's hospital, where he was voluntarily receiving outpatient psychiatric treatment. This psychotherapist requested that the campus police become involved, and they briefly detained the student but released him when he appeared to be rational. The psychotherapist's superior, a psychiatrist, directed that no further action be taken to detain the student, although it had been concluded that he represented an actual threat to the girl's safety. Neither the girl nor her parents were warned of the predicted peril, in apparent conformity with the student's right to confidentiality. The student did not return to the university's hospital for treatment, but persuaded the girl's brother to share an apartment with him and waited for her to return from vacation, when he brutally killed her.

The principal claim brought against the mental health professionals by the victim's parents on behalf of her estate was that they were in breach of a duty owed her to give appropriate warning of the danger she faced. It was claimed that such warning should have been given to the victim or to her parents or others who would be concerned for her safety. To the allegation that her death resulted from the defendants' negligent failure to warn the victim or others likely to apprise her of the danger she faced from the defendants' patient, the defendants made several responses. They claimed that their duty of confidentiality precluded improper disclosure, that no duty was owed the stranger to the physician–patient relation, and that psychiatry possessed no predictive powers regarding dangerousness on which a duty to warn can reasonably be based.

Regarding the defendants' claim of professional confidentiality, the court was not unsympathetic but addressed competing public interests by observing,

We recognize the public interest in supporting effective treatment of mental illness and in protecting the rights of patients to privacy, and the consequent public importance of safeguarding the confidential character of psychotherapeutic communication. Against this interest, however, we must weigh the public interest in safety from violent assault.[5]

This conflict was resolved in favor of the immediate victim and prospectively in favor of future potential individual victims, the court concluding,

The public policy favoring protection of the confidential character of patient–psychotherapist communications must yield to the extent to which disclosure is essential to avert danger to others. The protective privilege ends where the public peril begins.[6]

It was recognized that when there is danger, not to an identifiable individual, but to undifferentiated persons in the community at large, the appropriate response may be institution of civil committal proceedings aimed to remove the dangerous person from circulation.

Regarding the defense that no duty of reasonable care is owed to third persons arising out of relations between physicians or psychotherapists and their patients, the court reviewed general principles of delictual liability and its own precedents to conclude that "such a relationship may support affirmative duties for the benefit of third persons."[7] The court cited with approval from an authoritatively authored law journal article inspired by the first hearing of the *Tarasoff* case (Fleming & Maximov, 1974, p. 1030) that

there now seems to be sufficient authority to support the conclusion that by entering into a doctor–patient relationship the therapist becomes sufficiently involved to assume some responsibility for the safety, not only of the patient himself, but also of any third person whom the doctor knows to be threatened by the patient.[8]

The court applied this principle not only to the subjective circumstances of the *Tarasoff* case, where it was specifically concluded that the patient presented an actual danger to the individual whom he eventually killed, but also to an objective standard of prediction to be observed by professionals as a class. It was observed that

when a therapist determines, *or pursuant to the standards of his profession should determine,* that his patient presents a serious danger of violence to another, he incurs an obligation to use reasonable care to protect the intended victim against such danger.[9]

This was related directly to the defendants' third contention, namely, that as psychiatrists and psychotherapists they had no professional capacity to predict dangerousness in individual cases and accordingly could discharge no legal duty founded on a professional skill in clinical prognosis. The *Tarasoff* case constitutes a landmark in the evolution of professional psychiatry, because the American Psychiatric Association (APA) presented the court with an *amicus curiae* brief citing numerous articles published in preceding years that indicated that therapists, in the present state of the art,[10] are unable to predict violent acts reliably; the brief urged the court to consider these articles correct. The brief contended, indeed, that therapists' forecasts tend to overpredict violence consistently and are more often wrong than right.[11] The court, in response, observed:

We recognize the difficulty that a therapist encounters in attempting to forecast whether a patient presents a serious danger of violence. Obviously we do not require that the therapist, in making that determination, render a perfect performance; the therapist need only exercise "that reasonable degree of skill, knowledge, and care ordinarily possessed and exercised by members of [that professional specialty] under similar circumstances."[12] Within the broad range of reasonable practice and treatment in which professional opinion and judgment may differ, the therapist is free to exercise his or her own best judgment without liability; proof, aided by hindsight, that he or she judged wrongly is insufficient to establish negligence.[13]

Having established that mere liability to professional error is not tantamount to professional negligence,[14] the court noted that the failure in the present case was claimed to lie not in prediction, but in negligent failure to warn once a prediction of danger had actually been made. The court repeated the principle of liability, however, in both subjective and objective professional terms, in observing that

once a therapist does in fact determine, or under applicable professional standards reasonably should have determined, that a patient poses a serious danger of violence to others, he bears a duty to exercise reasonable care to protect the foreseeable victim of that danger.[15]

Implications of the *Tarasoff* case

The court in the *Tarasoff* case was not blind to the conflicts and tensions the case posed between different interests within the community. Most notably at stake were the interests of psychiatric patients and potential patients, of psychiatrists, psychotherapists and other mental health professionals, and, for instance, of prospective victims of patients who may cause harm, including both individually identifiable and unidentifiable prospective victims. It was recognized that "the ultimate question of resolving the tension between the conflicting interests of patient and potential victim is one of social policy, not professional expertise" (citing from Fleming & Maximov, 1974, p. 1067). The risk of overprediction of violence addressed in the APA's brief was acknowledged, but the court concluded in the social assessment,

The risk that unnecessary warnings may be given is a reasonable price to pay for the lives of possible victims that may be saved.[16]

Appropriate social policy may be determined by courts of law, composed of judges alone or judges and juries when legislation and judicial discretion so provide, or by a multijudge tribunal at appellate levels of adjudication. Social policy is also determined, however, perhaps with more obvious democratic credentials, by enactments of legislatures. These may authorize involuntary detention of persons found by different tests to be dangerous to others or to themselves and may also impose liabilities on and grant immunities to various professional, institutional, and other actors in the field of detection and treatment of mentally abnormal persons.

Accordingly, responses to the prediction, overprediction, and predictive failures of dangerousness may appear to be conditioned by laws and court decisions founded on social policy rather than on the perceptions and preferences of any individual professional group. The claim by professional psychiatry, represented in the APA's brief, of inability to predict dangerousness may appear, not as a complete disclaimer of skill, but rather as a claim to a level of skill that is prone to unreliability and inaccuracy. This is a factor in the discharge of professional responsibility of which social policy expressed in law may take due account. The

Tarasoff case may indeed have been unsuitable as a basis for a professional disclaimer of any ability to predict danger, because on the facts of the case the prediction that was actually made proved unfortunately to be completely correct.

The *Tarasoff* decision is of distinctive significance in marking official recognition by professional psychiatry, in the brief submitted by the APA,[17] that practitioners possess only limited capacity to predict dangerousness accurately and that predictions are more often wrong than right. Implicitly recognized was the threat to individual liberty of the false positive result of clinical prognosis. The decision in the case has caused great turmoil in the profession, however, and has stimulated agonized responses of distress and alarm.[18] In a sense, this may have been anticipated. The APA's brief explained that psychiatrists overpredict danger in patients, and, responding to the same instincts and perhaps motives, they have overpredicted danger in the judgment from their duty to warn and the absence of confidentiality where identifiable third parties are at risk. In this, too, they may be expected to be more often wrong than right.[19]

The judgment has been of revolutionary impact on psychiatrists' and clinical psychologists' perceptions of their role and responsibilities in the United States, Canada, and beyond, but in Canada at least its spirit was echoed, without the same response of outrage and alarm, in a 1977 judgment of the Supreme Court. In *Wellesley Hospital v. Lawson*,[20] a psychiatric patient assessed as violent was permitted to escape secure custody within the hospital, whereupon he seriously assaulted another patient. The victim sued the hospital for negligence, and the hospital raised a defense under the Mental Health Act of Ontario,[21] which provides that "no action lies against any psychiatric facility or any officer, employee or servant thereof for a tort of any patient." The trial court dismissed the claim on this basis, but the court of appeal found a triable issue against the hospital. In the Supreme Court of Canada, it was confirmed that the action against the hospital was not for the tort of the patient in injuring the victim, but for the hospital's own tort of negligence in allowing a patient diagnosed as dangerous to have access to other persons unaware of the risk. The hospital was held liable.

The case may be distinguishable from *Tarasoff* in that hospitals more readily acknowledge the duty of care they owe to patients not only against their own negligence in treatment and in providing safe accommodation, but also against injury arising from negligent management of other patients regarding, for instance, the spread of infection. Public policy giving hospitals and their staff protection from liability for wrongs caused by patients themselves, and particularly psychiatric patients, is evident in the provision of the Ontario legislation affording hospital and staff immunity. The special relationship creating a hospital's own legal duty of care is more easily recognized regarding a patient than it was regarding the identifiable stranger who was the victim in *Tarasoff*. In another sense, however, the duty in *Tarasoff* may have been more obvious and compel-

ling that it was in *Lawson,* because in the California case it was predicted that
the patient was an actual severe danger to that very victim, whereas in the latter
case it was not predictable that the victim of injury would be Lawson. The duty
owed to Lawson as a hospital patient is distinguishable from the duty owed to a
patient, staff member, hospital volunteer, and, for instance, visitor, as the potential victim of a dangerous psychiatric patient's attack. The *Lawson* decision may
extend liability from protection of predicted identifiable victims to protection of
predictable but unidentifiable victims.

The *Lawson* decision was congruent with *Tarasoff* in establishing liability for
insufficient protection against danger at two levels, that is, the level of actual
knowledge of danger and the level of knowledge imputable from the reasonable
exercise of professional skill and judgment. The Supreme Court of Canada held
that the hospital was bound by a duty to supervise and to keep under reasonable
control patients the hospital knew *or ought to have known* to have violent propensities.[22] This reflects a distinction that can be drawn from the *Tarasoff* case,
upon which the majority of the court and a dissenting judge (Mosk, J.) differed.
The distinction can be expressed in terms of the narrow or clinical *Tarasoff*
principle and the broad or normative principle, which the majority approved.

The narrow principle imposes liability when there is an insufficient response
to danger actually predicted following a clinical assessment reached on the
professionally diagnosed circumstances of the case. The broad principle imposes
liability when danger ought to have been predicted as a matter of professional
judgment, whether or not it actually was in the particular case. In both *Tarasoff*
and *Lawson,* liability arose under the narrow principle, in that an actual prediction of danger was made. In both judgments, however, the courts imposed liability on both narrow and broad principles. The disclaimer by professional psychiatry of general capacity to predict danger as a matter of professional skill casts
doubt on whether the broad or normative basis of liability can be maintained. It
certainly compels some reassessment in terms of public policy of the role that
psychiatrists, psychotherapists, and other mental health professionals should
continue to play in forensic and extrajudicial legal decisions. The disclaimer may
render unworkable not only liability under the broad *Tarasoff* principle, but several legal institutions that have become based on the belief, once encouraged by
mental health professionals, that they possess the professional skill generally to
predict dangerousness.

The challenge to professionalism

Practitioners of professions are legally required to observe the standards of skill
of the discipline they practice and to apply reasonably the knowledge they profess. Professions are historically distinguished from other groupings of persons
who earn a livelihood by common means, such as trade associations, by their

required mastery of a branch of learning or science. One may add such attributes as their tendency to be primarily self-policing and to determine qualification to commence and continue practice in the public interest, as well as their possession of a binding code of ethics reinforced by legislated or informal disciplinary ma- chinery. Essential to professional status, however, is an obligation to master, maintain, and develop a body of learning not shared by others in the community. The scope of professional practice is governed by the scope of the learning pro- fessed.[23]

The challenge the *Tarasoff* case poses to mental health professionalism is that, if practitioners wish for relief from legal liability for failure to predict danger- ousness reliably, they must so define their professional skills as to exclude that predictive capacity and recognize the limitation this imposes on the scope of legitimate professional practice and claims to expertise. Courts will clearly not hold professionals to standards of performance they deny they possess the knowl- edge to achieve, nor require that they achieve the impossible. Courts will be guided by appropriate expert witnesses in determining the levels of learning and standards of competence members of a given profession claim a capacity to ex- ercise, and once such standards are established, members must expect to be held to them in their general professional practice.

Consideration of who psychiatric professionals may be touches on wider is- sues of group definition than concern the area of mental health alone. Clearly, psychiatrists come within and probably may be considered to lead the ranks of professionals involved, secure in their status as physicians. Clinical psycholo- gists, perhaps under the name of psychotherapists, would also seem to be af- fected professionals, as the *Tarasoff* decision accepted. The practice claimed to be psychotherapy may be undertaken by other than psychology graduates, how- ever, such as psychoanalysts qualified or trained to different levels. Psychiatric nurses may now work in some jurisdictions as primary therapists in outpatient clinics, community mental health centers, and independent practices. Nurses of appropriate qualifications, such as master's degree level, claim expertise in psy- chotherapeutic methodologies and act as independent psychotherapists (e.g., Kjervik, 1981). Whether psychiatric social workers are professionals may be governed by the legal exclusiveness of their right to use that description and the means by which recruits to their ranks are qualified, registered, monitored, and, for instance, disciplined. The same may be said of educational psychologists working in schools and of marriage, family, and child counselors. Similarly, whether psychiatric ward orderlies, correctional officers, and others involved in administering care to and restraints on the mentally impaired hold themselves out to employees and the public as professionals depends on the special knowl- edge they profess to exercise and the same legal and administrative elements that constitute the legal status of psychiatric social workers.

Although expert witnesses are necessary to inform a court of the standards of performance of which particular professionals claim to be capable, the courts have an independent role in determining what level of professed skill has to be applied in a given relationship. In *Tarasoff*, the court followed the normal rule of expecting exercise of "that reasonable degree of skill, knowledge, and care ordinarily possessed and exercised by members of [that professional specialty] under similar circumstances."[24] A higher standard is expected of specialists than of general practitioners within a profession (see Picard, 1978, pp. 98–105). A professional performing below the degree of skill, knowledge, and care determined by this means may find it difficult to escape legal liability in negligence. Because the courts have a residual role to reinforce the professional duty of care, however, it does not follow that a practitioner who conforms to the customary standards of professional peers will necessarily avoid legal liability. The courts underwrite the expectation that professed skills will be appropriately rendered to those on whose behalf professional services are engaged.

This legal principle is acknowledged in Canada[25] but is most clearly illustrated in a 1974 case in Washington State. In *Helling v. Carey*,[26] a young woman attended an ophthalmologist for a routine examination, and the professional neither conducted nor advised a glaucoma test because there was no evidence that it was specifically indicated. The woman later suffered permanent damage to her sight from this cause and claimed that there was professional negligence in the failure to conduct or recommend the test. The defendant argued that it was general practice among professional peers in the locality and adjacent regions not to include such a test in a routine examination of a person under the age of 40 unless it was specifically indicated, and the court accepted the evidence that a glaucoma test was, indeed, not generally included in such routine examinations. Nevertheless, the court found that there had been professional negligence, because the patient, and by inference similar patients in the area, were entitled to a higher standard of care than the profession was apparently in the practice of rendering. The court explained that a patient attending such a routine examination expects to be informed of such tests as the glaucoma test, that is, tests that are reliable, safe, inexpensive, and capable of reducing the risk of major disablement. The test was well within the profession's capacity to perform and was the very service patients expect to be available. If there are many tests that conform to this description but the expense of having them all would be sizable, the decision as to which tests will be conducted and which will be declined should be made, not by the professional acting alone, but by the patient with the assistance of the professional's knowledge and judgment.

It is evident that if legal negligence is constituted by falling below legally set standards, and if professions were to enjoy exclusive power to determine their own standards of performance, they might have a self-serving incentive to set their standards lower than would serve the public interest. Accordingly, courts will monitor standards, on the incidence of litigation. Courts are limited in the setting of standards, however, to those that a profession is capable of achieving and will not demand exercise of skills not professed to be achievable by those qualified within the profession. Although courts, especially in the United States, appear to be increasingly accommodating of professional malpractice claims not only in medicine but also in law, social work, education, and, for instance, spiritual counseling (see Bergman, 1981; Ericsson, 1981), they determine standards, under the guidance of expert testimony, within limits of what professions claim they can achieve.[27]

Members of professions must in principle live up to their own claims of skills. Because professional psychiatry has now downgraded its professed skill in the clinical prediction of dangerousness, the broader principle of liability identified in *Tarasoff* and *Lawson,* namely, that appropriate responses must be made not only to patients actually predicted to be dangerous but also to those who pursuant to the standards of the profession ought to be known or predicted to be dangerous, loses much of its force. This limitation of claimed professional capacity protects members against unrealistic demands of their performance. It also presents new issues of public policy, however, because a marked degree of public reliance has come to be placed on professional possession of this predictive capacity, as evidenced in professionals' court appearances as expert witnesses.

Public reliance on professional prediction of dangerousness

There are many areas of legal activity in which mental health professionals have come to play a significant and perhaps decisive role because of their own claims or the acceptance by others that they possess a special capacity to predict dangerousness. The major areas of such activity are reviewed in the following sections.

Involuntary civil committal

Mental health legislation in Ontario reflects a movement observed to have occurred generally in North America and in a number of jurisdictions beyond (see Curran & Harding, 1978; Weissbourd, 1982) of allowing involuntary detention of persons who have not been convicted of criminal offenses only on the ground that they have been reliably found to be dangerous.

Before 1967, legislation in Ontario permitted a person's involuntary and indefinite confinement on certification by two physicians that the person was "mentally ill," meaning "suffering from such a disorder of the mind that he requires care, supervision and control for his own protection or welfare, or for the protection of others."[28] This "protection and welfare" indication for denial of liberty was tightened in 1967 to be based on a criterion of safety. Legislation in that year allowed a person's involuntary civil detention "in the interests of his own safety or the safety of others."[29] Detention could be based on the certificate of one physician, but of only 30 days' duration, only continued detention being subject to due process protections and open to initial and periodic reviews. This "safety" indication for committal to detention for psychiatric assessment proved to be open to many interpretations and possibilities of abuse, and in 1978 the indication was further refined to concentrate on a "dangerousness" indication for civil committal.[30] Section 9(1) of the Mental Health Act[31] now provides that:

where a physician examines a person and has reasonable cause to believe that the person,

(a)   has threatened or attempted or is threatening or attempting to cause bodily harm to himself;

(b)   has behaved or is behaving violently towards another person or has caused or is causing another person to fear bodily harm from him; or

(c)   has shown or is showing a lack of competence to care for himself,

and if in addition the physician is of the opinion that the person is apparently suffering from mental disorder of a nature or quality that likely will result in,

(d)   serious bodily harm to the person;

(e)   serious bodily harm to another person; or

(f)   imminent and serious physical impairment of the person,

the physician may make application in the prescribed form for a psychiatric assessment of the person.

By Section 10(1), information upon oath may be brought before a justice of the peace that a person satisfies criterion (a), (b), or (c), and if in addition the justice has reasonable cause to hold the belief identified in criterion (d), (e), or (f), the justice may issue an order for assessment by a physician. Similarly, by Section 11, a constable or peace officer who observes a person acting in a manner that in a normal person would be disorderly, who has reasonable cause to hold belief (a), (b), or (c), and who in addition forms the opinion identified in condition (d), (e), or (f) and considers that it would be dangerous to refer the matter to a justice of the peace under Section 10 may take the person in custody to an appropriate place for assessment by a physician.

Accordingly, the power a physician has to form an opinion to refer a person for psychiatric assessment is shared by a justice of the peace acting judicially and a police constable acting administratively. Because the professional reliability of a physician's opinion may be doubted, particularly since the physician forming the opinion may not specialize in psychiatry, it is instructive to note the parallel existence of comparable powers in the judiciary and police acting in their official capacities. These alternatives may provide models worthy of promotion.

The assessment for which a person is detained must be conducted "forthwith" after receipt of a person from a justice of the peace or a police officer[32] and within 120 hours of the application for assessment by a physician.[33] Assessment may result in further involuntary detention if the attending physician forms the opinion that the person is suffering from mental disorder of a nature or quality that likely will result in

(i) serious bodily harm to the person

(ii) serious bodily harm to another person, or

(iii) imminent and serious physical impairment of the person, unless the person remains in the custody of a psychiatric facility.[34]

This reinforces the significance of the dangerousness test to modern civil commitment.

The duty to warn

The narrow principle in *Tarasoff,* that when an actual prediction of danger to an identified person is made, an appropriate response may be to warn the potential victim or a suitable other person, warrants further attention. *Tarasoff* was concerned with the duty owed to the potential victim, but it may be noted in the case that, had a warning been given, this might have protected not only the victim from being killed, but also the patient from becoming a killer and enduring all of the consequences of that status. Accordingly, the warning response to actual prediction of dangerousness might discharge duties to both potential victim and patient.

It may be asked whether simply warning a potential victim of danger is therapeutically or legally sufficient, from the perspective of either the victim or the patient. Wexler (1981, p. 168, especially) has argued that violence-prone patients who feel hostility toward particular individuals, such as spouses or lovers, could be more effectively treated not individually but with some form of group therapy, including the presence of the potential victim whose behavior may trigger the patient's hostility.[35] If the target of hostility is a major political figure or a person such as a movie star or starlet who becomes the focus of an abnormal passion, one cannot expect that person's collaboration in the patient's therapy. Homicidal passion is more frequently directed, however, against family members and others with whom potential assailants have shared intense emotional relations.[36] The tendency of victims to precipitate their own injury and their inability or unwillingness to perceive the danger they cause themselves may support the view that an appropriate response to prediction of such danger may be not a mere warning, but an offer of individual therapy or joint counseling with the potential assailant, in order to attempt to resolve the dangerous disharmony generated within the relationship. The possible protection that psychiatrists and psychotherapists can thereby offer patients and their potential victims is dependent, of course, on their capacity to predict dangerousness in individual cases. If Wexler's perception were to find acceptance as doctrine, however, the expectation of seeking to involve potential victims who have been in close relationships with patients in group (meaning twin) therapy might become standard.

Criminal process

The roles of mental health professionals in drafting and contesting presentence reports and in the conduct of sentence hearings and their similar roles in bail proceedings and at hearings of parole boards require no elaboration. The functions of sentence upon criminal conviction are several and include both retrospective and prospective aspects. The prospective component of sentence is concerned with the likelihood of rehabilitation, of recurrence of offending, and of future dangerousness. Protection of members of the public in both individual and collective senses is an often invoked obligation of the courts and of parole boards. Accordingly, the assistance of mental health professionals in decision making based on estimates of offenders' future behavior is welcomed by courts and parole boards. Despite professional psychiatry's downgrading of claims to predictive skills, mental health professionals continue to participate significantly in these predictive exercises, although prognoses now tend to be presented with built-in limits and to be expressed with circumspection (see, e.g., Dix, 1978).

The part of criminal process that is most severely undercut by the recognition of unreliability of professional predictions of dangerousness is the part that was founded on and remains critically dependent on the credibility of such predictions. Part 21 of Canada's Criminal Code,[37] for instance, is entitled "Dangerous Offenders"; before 1977 the title was "Dangerous Sexual Offenders" (see Klein, 1976). It provides for indeterminate sentence in a penitentiary of offenders whose past conduct renders them eligible for an application at sentence for them to be found dangerous offenders, and who, upon the evidence of named professionals, are so found. The offender must have been convicted of a serious personal injury offense, defined[38] as (a) an indictable offense (other than treasons and murder)[39] involving the use or attempted use of violence or conduct endangering or likely to endanger life or safety or inflicting or likely to inflict severe psychological damage, and (b) sexual offenses ranging from sexual assault to aggravated sexual assault.

Regarding offenses in category (a), an offender may be found a dangerous offender and receive indeterminate sentence on the basis of evidence establishing[40]

(i) a pattern of repetitive behaviour . . . showing a failure to restrain his behaviour and a likelihood of his causing death or injury to other persons, or inflicting severe psychological damage upon other persons, through failure in the future to restrain his behaviour,

(ii) a pattern of persistent aggressive behaviour . . . showing a substantial degree of indifference on the part of the offender as to the reasonably foreseeable consequences to other persons of his behaviour,

or,

(iii) any behaviour by the offender . . . that is of such brutal nature as to compel the conclusion that his behaviour in the future is unlikely to be inhibited by normal standards of behavioural restraint.

Regarding sexual offenses defined in category (b), an offender may be classified as dangerous if, by his record of conduct in any sexual matter,

he has shown a failure to control his sexual impulses and a likelihood of his causing injury, pain or other evil to other persons through failure in the future to control his sexual impulses.[41]

An application requires consent of the provincial attorney general and at least 7 days' prior notice to the accused.[42] It shall be heard and determined "by the court without a jury,"[43] and "the court *shall* hear the evidence of at least two psychiatrists and all other evidence . . . including the evidence of any psychologist or criminologist called as a witness."[44] Of the two psychiatrists the judge is obliged to hear, one shall be nominated by the prosecution and one by the offender.[45]

These proceedings are completely dependent on the expert testimony of at least two psychiatrists,[46] the apparent inferences being that psychiatrists are experts on dangerousness, that they can reliably predict dangerousness, and that dangerousness cannot reliably be predicted without psychiatric testimony. Professional psychiatry, as represented in the APA's brief in *Tarasoff*, now appears to contend, however, that none of these inferences is true. Psychiatrists disclaim expertise in such prediction, deny reliability of their prognoses, and indeed positively assert their inherent unreliability,[47] and courts have recognized that "psychiatrists are not uniquely qualified to predict dangerous behaviour and are, in fact, less accurate in their predictions than other professionals"[48] (Ennis & Litwack, 1974, p. 712) Accordingly, the entire philosophical and empirical foundations of the dangerous offender provisions of the Canadian Criminal Code would seem to have been removed. Part 21 of the Criminal Code stands as no more than an altar to discredited mythology on which offenders whom psychiatrists dislike[49] are arbitrarily[50] sacrificed to indeterminate imprisonment.

Another feature of Part 21 of the code is its recognition of "criminologists." These persons are not defined, but by canons of statutory construction (notably the *noscitur a sociis* or the *ejusdem generis* rule) they may appear in the same class as psychiatrists and psychologists. Because by negative definition they are neither, however, one may speculate that they are less qualified in the disciplines of psychiatry and psychology than those who are qualified, whose own predictions are not reliable. Ironically, they may be the "other professionals," perhaps, such as psychiatric social workers and correctional officers, whose predictions have been judicially recognized to be more accurate.[51] Recognition of their right to appear as expert witnesses confirms the belief underlying this procedure that dangerousness can be predicted by experts.

The fact that an application must be decided "by the court without a jury"[52] shows that "dangerousness" is determined as a matter of law and not as a matter of fact, because in jury trials judges determine the law and juries resolve issues of fact. This may offer a helpful analytic approach to the "dangerousness" concept,[53] but because the credibility of opposing expert witnesses is in question and much turns upon presented details of the offender's immediate offense and particularly evidence of past behavior on the basis of which future behavior may be anticipated, it may appear that an application raises issues on which a jury's assessment is no less valuable than that of a judge.

Policing functions

Indirect. Mental health professionals discharge policing functions indirectly by giving information to the regular police force about matters that, and persons who, may endanger the peace that police are dedicated to preserving and violation of which the police investigate for purposes of prosecution. In *Tarasoff* it was considered that involving the police when dangerousness was predicted might well be an appropriate and legitimate response,[54] particularly if the potential victim were unidentified or would probably be an unidentifiable person drawn at random. If the potential victim were identified or reasonably identifiable, however, the duty to warn that person or a suitable other especially concerned for the person's welfare was preferred, as is consistent with modern principles of seeking the least restrictive alternative means of mental health management. Police believe that disclosure is not merely appropriate when danger threatens, but that it should be mandatory. They also commonly urge their right of access to psychiatric and other data to predict and thereby deter violence and to detect offenders after the event.[55] In the conflict between security of individuals and the public, on the one hand, and liberty including confidentiality of the individual, on the other, the police understandably promote their vision of security.[56]

The police acquire a strong incentive to protect the identities of their informants, including mental health professionals who supply information about persons believed to be dangerous and persons who have apparently been involved in violence. Police responses to the receipt of such information are governed by their convictions regarding its reliability. Police, like psychiatrists, however, are prone to overpredict the danger presented by a suspected source, and they may add their own overreactions to mental health professionals' overreactions under the justification of serving security and minimizing the risk of victimization of innocent persons. Judicial support has been given at high levels to police protection of identities of informants warning of danger.

In October 1981, the Supreme Court of Canada reflected a 1978 decision in an English case in the House of Lords upholding the immunity of agencies discharging policing functions from having to disclose names of informants who gave them data relevant to future danger. The Canadian case arose when the Royal Commission of Inquiry into Confidentiality of Health Records in Ontario (Commissioner: Mr. Justice Krever) asked the Royal Canadian Mounted Police (RCMP) to reveal names of physicians who had supplied them with information about patients without the patients' consent. The Commissioner's request was designed, not to lead to preliminary proceedings for breach of confidentiality, but to permit questioning of informants to ascertain whether their communications were voluntary or whether they had been coerced or induced by improper means. The RCMP declined to reveal informants' identities, supporting nondisclosure through three arguments:

(i) they needed the information to assist in enforcing federal narcotic control legislation;

(ii) they needed psychiatric information about certain patients who might pose a threat to foreign dignitaries and other prominent individuals; and

(iii) they needed the information to assist in combatting subversion, espionage and terrorism.[57]

A majority of the court held that "public interest immunity"[58] protected the claim to nondisclosure advanced by the RCMP, because police informer privilege is recognized in law; it was noted that the privilege was applied in the 1978 House of Lords case to protective agencies other than the police. Furthermore, the majority found that

the foundation for the existence of this rule of law, which evolved in respect of the field of criminal investigation, is even stronger in relation to the function of the police in protecting national security. A large number of the instances in which, in the present case, it was sought to obtain from the police the names of their informants concerned police investigation into potential violence against officers of the State, including heads of State. These investigations were admittedly proper police functions. The rule of law which protects against the disclosure of informants in the police investigation of crime has even greater justification in relation to the protection of national security against violence and terrorism.[59]

Thus, it was recognized that police and others may protect identities of informants who give them information predicting danger, because such agencies require and may rely on information they receive. The immunity from disclosure applies not only if the information is incorrect, unreliable, and negligent, but also if it is malicious and intended to deceive. The Supreme Court majority cited the 1978 House of Lords judgment on this point. The English case concerned a person who untruly informed the National Society for Prevention of Cruelty to Children[60] (NSPCC) that the plaintiff had abused her child. The plaintiff wanted to sue the informant, but the NSPCC refused to reveal the informant's identity. The plaintiff sued the NSPCC for negligence in failing to investigate the complaint properly and sought disclosure of all documents related to it, including those revealing the informant's identity. The NSPCC applied for an order protecting that identity. The House of Lords unanimously held that the order should be issued, because of the importance of the rule of law protecting names of those who inform agencies discharging police and comparable functions. It was recognized that those who inform of predicted danger may also misinform and overinform. The House of Lords observed, however, that

the rule can operate to the advantage of the untruthful or malicious or revengeful or self-interested or even demented police informant as much as of one who brings information from a high-minded sense of civic duty. Experience seems to have shown that though the resulting immunity from disclosure can be abused the balance of public advantage lies in generally respecting it.[61]

Thus, on grounds of public policy, policing agencies are entitled to protect the identities of those such as mental health professionals who inform them of predicted danger, however unreliable the prediction may be. Those giving the information do not thereby acquire legal immunity of their own from legal liability, for possible breach of duties under public hospital legislation or for defamation, for instance,[62] but they are secure in the knowledge that the policing agencies can keep the assurances they give to protect their identities. The inherent unreliability of dangerousness predictions may in time compel judicial reassessment of the experience showing that the balance of public advantage lies in respecting the protected status of such predictions, but a judiciary preoccupied by considerations of security seems unlikely to review the rule of protected communication.

Direct. Mental health professionals have the legal power to discharge police functions of the state by acting directly against those they assess to be dangerous. This matter was fully reviewed in the U.S. courts in the case of *Rogers v. Okin,*[63] a lengthy and complex civil rights class action. The relevant issues for the present purposes were whether involuntarily detained mental health patients can be involuntarily treated and in particular under what circumstances state officials may forcibly administer antipsychotic drugs to restrain mental health patients without violating constitutional protections of personal bodily and mental integrity.[64] Simply stated, the U.S. Court of Appeals concluded that such involuntary administration of drugs could not be justified as a therapeutic measure because competent patients and guardians of the incompetent have a legal right to refuse risk-bearing antipsychotic drugs,[65] but it may be justified as a police measure undertaken by mental health professionals.[66]

The court's decision distinguished between two bases of treatment of persons involuntarily detained in state-run hospitals as a result of mental illness, namely, the *parens patriae* power and the police power. The historic *parens patriae* power arose as part of the sovereign's conscientious duty to protect the weak and the vulnerable, such as infants and the mentally impaired. It is a benign power, used to protect and advance the bodily, material, and spiritual welfare of the disabled. The court cited earlier judgments[67] for the proposition that

the *sine qua non* for the state's use of its *parens patriae* power as justification for the forceful administration of mind-affecting drugs is a determination that the individual to whom the drugs are to be administered lacks the capacity to decide for himself whether he should take the drugs.[68]

It was found, however, that the law of the state concerned, Massachusetts, contained nothing to show that findings of patients' mental illness were equivalent to findings of their incompetence to determine for themselves whether commitment and treatment would be in their own best interest. In fact, that law provided a proceeding separate from that resulting in involuntary committal in order to determine the issue, which must be regarded as a separate issue, of competency. This is consistent with the basis of detention being dangerousness, not treatability or incompetence.[69] The court concluded that

the commitment decision itself is an inadequate predicate to forcible administration of drugs to an individual where the purported justification for that action is the state's *parens patriae* power.[70]

The proposition that involuntarily committed persons are necessarily incompetent and that they may accordingly be treated without their consent was thereby rejected. Even if they are independently shown to be incompetent, moreover, so that they fall under the disposition of others, it does not follow that those given substituted or surrogate consent power over incompetents can use the power arbitrarily or in service to their individual preferences. They must instead use their power as would the incompetent persons were they to be competent.[71] This limitation is implicit in the *parens patriae* power.

In contrast, the police power may be applied directly against the mentally ill, in the overtly stated interests of others. The court recognized that certain drugs may present risks to those taking them but that not administering them may present risks of danger to others. Accordingly, the involved professionals must engage in risk-to-benefit calculation and reach an individualized decision specific to the patient liable to be affected, the nature and extent of the risk of dangerousness to others that the patient seems to present, and the comparable risk of receiving the drug. Permitting involuntary and possibly forcible administration of antipsychotic drugs to those competent to refuse to take them, the court stated that

the state's purpose in administering drugs forcibly must be to further its police power interests, i.e., the decision must be the result of a determination that the need to prevent violence in a particular situation outweighs the possibility of harm to the medicated individual.[72]

The court repeated that "medication cannot be forcibly administered solely for treatment purposes absent a finding of incompetency"[73] and explored the elements of procedural due process that have to attend the determination to exercise the police power. Underlying this elaboration, however, was the recognition that mental health professionals may impose risk-bearing drug administrations on nonconsenting competent persons under a police power predicated on professional ability to predict violence and dangerousness to others. Psychiatrists, psychologists, and others are entrusted with the power to impose policing by pharmacology.

Public policy in the face of clinical unpredictability of dangerousness

It has been seen that many powers have become vested in mental health professionals on the basis of the capacity to predict dangerousness in individual cases, which they have come to deny they possess. We must therefore address the issue of the responses public policy should make to public and legal reliance on this once supposed but now disclaimed capacity. Two closely related proposals may be advanced, the incidents of which will be considered in the context of areas of public reliance on trustworthy predictive skills. These are (a) that "dangerousness" be recognized as a legal status as opposed to a psychiatric condition and (b) that dangerousness be determined by due process of law in adequately conducted hearings.

"Dangerousness" as a legal status

Dangerousness cannot be predicted by mental health professionals as a clinical prognosis with adequate reliability, but the concept of dangerousness concerns an anxious public, which requires that fear of danger receive a protective response. This can be found in recognizing dangerousness, not as a psychiatric condition or prognosis, but as a legal status attaching to a person at a given time with potentially enduring consequences. The models for this legal concept are the concepts in criminal law of "insanity" and "disease of the mind" that causes insanity. The highest courts have recognized that the concept of insanity based on disease of the mind is a concept of law,[74] to be determined by a judge. The concept includes a substantial medical component, and medical expert witnesses are almost invariably involved in its determination, with psychologists also playing an influential role. Its nature and basis are determined, however, by a judge, and members of a jury may reach an independent assessment of whether the legally defined elements of the status were actually present at the time of a given incident, taking into account their views of the defendant's past behavior and present demeanor, as well as expert medical testimony and that of lay witnesses. The legal status of insanity and of disease of the mind are progressively clarified, refined, and developed by jurisprudence and judgments in response to medical and psychological data, mental health professional prognostic capacitities, and also public perceptions.

Courts have already observed the exclusive legal character of the condition of dangerousness. In *State v. Hudson* late in 1979, for instance, the Supreme Court of New Hampshire noted:

Nor must a finding of dangerousness be founded only upon psychiatric or other expert medical testimony. The condition of dangerousness is not a medical concept but rather a legal one.[75]

Accordingly, the importance attached to psychiatric predictive evidence may be downgraded, consistently with its inherent unreliability, and such factors as immediate past behavior[76] and its perceived causes and their likelihood of recurrence may be assessed by judge and jury with confidence in their own predictive capabilities.

Outside the setting of the courts, the duty to warn of the legal condition of dangerousness would remain only on the narow *Tarasoff* principle, that is, when an actual prediction were made. The duty here may be owed no less to the patient than to the potential victim, because protection of the latter may also protect the former, and a warning may be the least invasive means of protection. The broad or normative principle of *Tarasoff* could not be maintained, because this requires a mental health professional to determine dangerousness "pursuant to the standards of his profession."[77] Although one may be said to be presumed to know the law, recognition that the concept of dangerousness originates and finds its substance in law may weaken the perception that its determination is a matter of observing mental health professional standards. Professionals are expected to be competent in the concepts of their own disciplines, such as the concept of mental illness, but they cannot be held legally liable for not acting in accordance with concepts arising and developing within another profession and branch of learning. Mental health professionals who may be legally liable for failure to diagnose mental illness, for instance, would not be so liable for failure or inability to diagnose "insanity" or "disease of the mind." Their role in determining these conditions, if any, is as expert witnesses to medical fact and opinion whose testimony is at best influential but is not in itself decisive of the legal issue.[78] If "dangerousness" were to acquire the same status, there would be comparable protection for mental health professionals who failed to predict it in clinical assessments. This would be scientifically appropriate, because such prediction is no longer claimed to be a clinical professional skill.

"Dangerousness" determination by due process of law

The principle that the legal status or condition of dangerousness should be determined in accordance with due process of law is not only internally consistent, but consistent with other areas of preventive intervention, in both civil law and criminal law. It has been seen that civil committal may be triggered under, for instance, Ontario's Mental Health Act[79] by one of three procedures. Under Section 9(1), a physician may take an initiative to commit for assessment, which must be undertaken within 120 hours of involuntary detention.[80] Alternatively, however, a police officer may take a person behaving in a disorderly way to an appropriate place for assessment, and in particular, by Section 10(1) of the act, information on oath may be presented in court before a justice of the peace that a person has shown behavior threatening bodily harm (or lack of competence in self-care). If the justice then finds reasonable cause on the evidence to believe that the person is apparently suffering from mental disorder that likely will result in serious bodily harm (or imminent and serious physical impairment of the person), the justice may order medical assessment.[81]

The attending physician shall observe and examine a person brought for assessment and may admit the person to hospital as an involuntary patient if finding mental disorder that is likely to result in serious bodily harm (or imminent and serious physical impairment of the person). Immediately upon becoming an involuntary patient, the patient or any person on the patient's behalf may appeal to an appropriately constituted review board[82] against involuntary admission, and the same right exists upon periodic renewal of a certificate of involuntary detention. Furthermore, whether or not objection to detention is initiated by or on behalf of the patient, automatic periodic reviews of involuntary detention are conducted by the review board. Under the general law and under habeas corpus provisions, there may be recourse to the courts against decisions of review boards.[83]

If dangerousness were a reliably predictable medical or psychiatric condition, initial intervention through a physician and a psychiatric assessment would be justifiable, with courts of law available for subsequent resort to ensure that procedures of psychiatric detention had been lawfully used. If dangerousness were to be recognized, however, as a legal status or condition, it would be appropriate for initial involuntary intervention with persons suspected of being dangerous to be undertaken through courts, which would consider medical and other evidence.[84] This has always been so in the field of preventive criminal justice, which has existed since antiquity, having roots that are more anthropological than merely historical.[85] Restraints on feared violence may be imposed, at the cost of loss of freedom of persons who have not violated the law, only by judicial order.

The power of a justice of the peace to bind over a person to be of good behavior was first expressed in legislation in what is now known as the Justice of the Peace Act, 1361,[86] but this formalized earlier practice. The power is now expressed in Canada[87] in the Criminal Code,[88] Section 745(1), which provides that

any person who fears that another person will cause personal injury to him or his wife or child or will damage his property may lay an information before a justice.

The justice shall then cause the parties to appear before an appropriate court of law, where the informant may adduce evidence of the grounds of fear. If the case is made, the court may order the defendant to give specified undertakings to be of good conduct for a period of up to 12 months, and if the defendant fails or refuses to observe the conditions offered, there may be commitment to prison for a term not exceeding 12 months.[89] Breach of an order made under this provision is punishable as a summary offense.[90] This sanction would clearly be inadequate for conduct such as occurred in *Tarasoff*, but had a warning of apprehended danger been given in time to the victim or her parents and had a court proceeding of this nature followed, the court might have imposed conditions such as compliance with psychiatric treatment and living away from the victim's brother, which might have prevented the tragic incident.

It may accordingly be proposed that involuntary committal to a mental health facility of a person who has not committed an offense should be lawful, not on a physician's reference to a psychiatrist, whose prognosis of dangerousness may cause a person's loss of liberty, which may eventually be open to challenge in a court, but only on initial resort to a court of law. Both civil and criminal legislation in force provide elements of procedure that may be drawn together to provide a procedural model.

The immediate frame of reference is child protection legislation, illustrated by Ontario's Child Welfare Act.[91] When it is suspected that a child is in need of protection, an appropriate person or officer may apply to a family court judge for an order requiring the person in charge of the child to produce the child at a judicial hearing at a stated place and time. The merits of the suspicion are then determined in judicial proceedings. Alternatively, when the fear is of immediate danger, the child may be seized without warrant, and with the use of reasonable force if necessary, and detained in a place of safety until the matter can be brought to family court. Court proceedings must be brought as soon as is practicable, and in any event within 5 days of the child being detained, or the child must be returned to the person having charge of the child immediately before the detention, unless that person agrees to another arrangement. An alternative to this means of taking into custody a child at apparent risk is for a person to lay an information on oath before a justice, who may issue a warrant authorizing a police officer or other specified person to search for the child and to take the child for detention in a place of safety. As before, the child must then be brought before the court within 5 days for determination of need of protection or be released. The child may have legal representation in any court proceedings, and under given conditions legal representation shall be provided by direction of the court.

This basic model may be translated for application to civil committal. When it is suspected that a person is dangerous, a physician, psychotherapist, or other person may apply to an appropriate court[92] to set a time and place for a hearing, when the merits of the suspicion may be determined. A judge may make an order remanding the suspected person for psychiatric assessment if desirable[93] and adjourn the proceedings for a brief assessment period. Alternatively, when immediate danger is feared, the suspected person may be seized without warrant, and with the use of reasonable force if necessary,[94] and detained, restrained,[95] and assessed in a place of safety until the matter can be brought to court. Court proceedings must begin as soon as is practicable, and in any event within 5 days of detention,[96] or the person must be released. Alternatively, an information may be laid before a justice, as provided in Section 10 of the present Mental Health Act,[97] who may issue a warrant for the suspected person to be taken to a place of assessment and to court for an appropriate hearing within 5 days if the assessment does not lead to earlier release. Upon accepting an applicant's evidence from the assessment that the suspected person is dangerous, the judge may make an appropriate order for detention and, subject to prior notification and the person's representations, perhaps for nonconsensual treatment.[98] Detention might be for finite periods, subject to renewal after an appropriate hearing.

Judicial proceedings in this form would depart from present regular means of imposing involuntary detention for assessment and subsequently, in affording suspected parties legal representation, early access to information of the evidence and reports to be used against them, means of securing expert and other evidence to be used on their own behalf, judicially reasoned decisions, and access to the regular means of appeal. Those suspected of dangerousness need not be prejudiced by adverse publicity because family courts regularly protect the identities of vulnerable persons in proceedings before them, for instance, by preventing the publication of names and other identifying information. Rights to enter mental facilities as voluntary patients would not be impaired, and after judicially approved detention consequent upon adverse psychiatric assessment, patients would preserve rights of periodic invited and spontaneous review. Furthermore, authorities would retain their present powers of emergency intervention to prevent danger from imminent violence and could present their explanations after the fact.

It may be objected that judicialization of civil committal in this form would impair mental health care and treatment and tie up the scarce and expensive resource of mental health professionals in court preparation and proceedings. It may also seem that presenting the pattern of committal as simply advancing resort to the courts ahead of where it is available under present circumstances is distortion of the present balance of extrajudicial and judicial decision making. Once it is recognized, however, that dangerousness is to be regarded as a legal status or condition, and the profession's own evidence is accepted that mental health practitioners have no reliable means to predict dangerousness in individual cases, it follows that free and nonoffending persons should not be denied their liberty with fewer due process protections. Considering the protections afforded criminal defendants before they forfeit liberty, it may be that nonoffenders who may be mentally ill should be afforded nothing less. Indeed, it may further be claimed that, in judicial proceedings of this nature, the required standard of proof of the applicants' case should be not the regular civil standard of proof on a balance of probabilities but, because loss of freedom is involved, the criminal standard of proof beyond reasonable doubt. A compromise, based on the consideration that involuntary detention may save the detainee from the consequences of an awful act and offer a prospect of advisable treatment, may consist of the standard of requiring "clear and convincing" evidence of dangerousness.[99]

It has already been observed that, in the face of professional disclaimers of reliable clinical predictive skills, dangerous offender provisions imposing indeterminate preventive detention are difficult to maintain. Strong arguments have been presented for many years that provisions such as appear in Part 21 of Canada's Criminal Code should be repealed, both for their doctrinal fallacies and for the practical inequities and oppression to which they so often contribute (see, e.g., Price, 1970, including extensive references to earlier literature; Schiffer, 1978, pp. 263–87; Webster & Dickens, 1983). If they are to be preserved in any form, however, two amendments in particular would seem to be required. First, notwithstanding the "scientific" pretenses of the determination to be made, involving psychiatrists, psychologists, and "criminologists," the key facts are related to the offender's past record of behavior. Because the predictive significance of this can be as reliably interpreted by others as by mental health professionals, the role of the jury should be preserved when trial has been by jury. The judge should inform the jury of what factors and features may constitute dangerousness in law, as in the case of insanity, and it should be for the jury to assess whether the accused's evidenced behavior, in conjunction with other evidence including that of professional opinion, satisfies the tests set. Second, the obligation to call two psychiatrists should be removed and a discretion be given to each side. Apart from giving the parties rights instead of obligations, this would preserve the system even if psychiatrists were to decline in the future to participate in an exercise in which they recognize that they have no reliable skills.

Far more important than the role of mental health professionals in dangerous offender proceedings, although scarcely less contentious, is their role in sentence hearings and before parole boards. It would be, perhaps, unduly repetitious to say why their function as predictors of dangerousness cannot be discharged. They may be able to contribute important information about an offender's apparent present disposition and attitudes to past events including the convicted offense. Interpretation of these data and its projection into the future do not require expert assessment. Mental health professionals may appear as experts in determining an offender's present characteristics, perhaps aiding a decision on whether they amount in law to dangerousness. Regarding the future, however, no expert role can be claimed, and mental health evidence may be regarded in much the same way as character evidence in indicating an offender's potential.

The role of mental health professionals in giving information to the police is comparable to that of other informants, although perhaps more credible regarding a potential dangerous offender's present disposition and maintenance of a profile or short-term syndrome objectively associated with immediate violence. Acquisition of a dangerous weapon, for instance, related to the pursuit of an obvious identified or unidentified person as likely victim, would clearly justify and even compel police involvement. If information is given in circumstances other than those calling for prompt intervention, however, whether in response to police solicitation or on spontaneous initiative, a condition should in principle be observed, which has come into recent recognition in related areas, that when police receive such a report and place it on file, they serve a standard form of notice on the person named.

An obvious exception to this principle exists when matters of espionage and national security are involved, although it would remain a matter of police judgment whether persons suspected of potential terrorism might be deterred by knowledge of police surveillance. When the notification principle is observed, furthermore, the identities of informants would remain protected, in accordance with doctrines approved at the highest judicial levels.[100] The general principle of disclosure as a feature of public policy draws its strength, however, from legislation rather than case law. Criminal Code provisions on the interception of private communications, by bugging of a telephone, for instance, require specified notification to the person affected.[101] Similarly, general freedom of information legislation and that applicable more selectively to commercial credit ratings records and comparable personal information data banks express the principle of the individual's right to disclosure.[102] At provincial levels, legislation such as Ontario's Child Welfare Act,[103] which creates a register of abused children, also entitles their adult guardians to notice of registration of their names,[104] and in the same spirit the Royal Commission of Inquiry into Confidentiality of Health Records in Ontario recommended that patients have access to their own medical files.[105] This would apply to psychiatric patients no less than others, but implementing legislation would establish procedures for exceptions to disclosure, perhaps comparable to those under the provincial Mental Health Act governing patient and other access to the medical record pursuant to a subpoena, order, direction, notice, or similar requirement.[106]

Implicit in the right to disclosure, often made explicit in implementing legislation, is the right to challenge, to correct errors of fact, and to present contradictory evidence. Whether an objection or appeal against an unfavorable and erroneous record is heard by a court or another tribunal such as a commissioner or standing ad hoc committee is a matter secondary to the governing principle. A person whom the police accept is dangerous should have the power to contest the psychiatric basis of the claim and to show to independent satisfaction that police acceptance of the status is not justified and that the adverse record or entry be destroyed or expunged.

Regarding the function of mental health professionals in direct policing of those determined to be dangerous, the court in *Rogers v. Okin* recognized that a legitimate protective and restraining role can be performed, including through recourse to forcible administration of antipsychotic drugs, within the limits of predictive powers. The court found, however, that constitutional protection against deprivation of liberty[107] positively required

the imposition of procedures whereby the necessary determinations can be made with due process.[108]

The court indicated that this requires, for example, the decision of a physician specific to the individual patient who is to be nontherapeutically medicated or otherwise managed. There was no further elaboration of detail – this was left to the lower court to which the case was remanded – but the court noted that the lower tribunal should

limit its own role to designing procedures for ensuring that the patients' interests in refusing antipsychotics are taken into consideration and that antipsychotics are not forcibly administered absent a finding by a qualified physician that those interests are outweighed in a particular situation and less restrictive alternatives are unavailable.[109]

It may be anticipated that a procedure so designed would find mental health professionals playing a highly visible role, but due process would require prior submission of reports to a representative of the patient. Whether this were a lawyer engaged by or on behalf of the patient, who would refer reports to a mental health professional also engaged in service to the patient's wishes, or a patients' rights officer or ombudsman in a psychiatric facility, would be governed by the urgency of the circumstances and the resources that could be devoted to them.

This narrow issue presents an instructive microcosm of the general issue on which to conclude. Once it is accepted that, as evidenced by the psychiatric brief in the *Tarasoff* case, reliable clinical predictions of dangerousness cannot be made by mental health professionals, any interference with the freedom of individuals and with their legal rights to autonomy and personal integrity can be justified only as an outcome of determinations made in accordance with due process of law. Such process may be conducted in courts or in other tribunals composed, perhaps, of persons other than lawyers but with an aggrieved person retaining the power to seek and possibly to compel judicial review of proceedings resulting in an invasive, inhibiting, or otherwise offensive conclusion. If, however, professional psychiatry and related mental health professions claim a reliability of predictive capacity that renders these due process protections against oppressive error unnecessary, then legal liability for the direct and forseeable consequences of falling below the professional standard of prediction that ought to be observed must be accepted.

Notes

1 See the section on criminal process under "Public Reliance on Professional Prediction of Dangerousness" regarding, for instance, Part 21 of the Criminal Code of Canada.

2 529 P.2d 553 (Superior Ct., Alameda Co., 1974).

3 (1976), 551 P.2d 334 (S.C. Cal.).

4 For reversal of the student's conviction for second-degree murder, on account of insanity, see *People v. Poddar* (1974), 518 P.2d 342 (S.C. Cal.).

5 See note 3, p. 346.

6 Ibid., p. 347; also see generally B. Dickens (1978).

7 See note 3, p. 343.

8 Ibid., p. 344.

9 Ibid., p. 340, per Tobriner, J. (emphasis added). The observation is repeated with minor word changes on p. 345; see n. 15.

10 The claim apparently was that mental health therapy is an art, as opposed to, for instance, a science.

11 See note 3, p. 344.

12 Citing *Bardessono v. Michels* (1970), 478 P.2d 480 at p. 438 (S.C. Cal).

13 See note 3, p. 345.

14 For another authoritative ruling that mere error of professional judgment is not tantamount to professional negligence, see the English House of Lords case of *Whitehouse v. Jordan*, [1981] 1 W.L.R. 246; [1981] 1 All E.R. 267, involving the use of forceps in childbirth associated with severe brain damage, in which a finding of negligence was reversed as being unfounded.

15 See note 3, p. 345.

16 Ibid., p. 346. The court added, "We would hesitate to hold that the therapist who is aware that his patient expects to attempt to assassinate the President of the United States would not be

obligated to warn the authorities because the therapist cannot predict with accuracy that his patient will commit the crime.''

17 A comparable *amicus curiae* brief was submitted by the American Psychiatric Association to the U.S. Supreme Court in the case of *Estelle v. Smith* (1981), 101 S.Ct. 1866, arguing against reliance upon psychiatrists' predictions on issues of dangerousness; see the discussion in Braley (1981).

18 It has also stimulated healthy professional reappraisal, of which the series of lectures generating this volume may be a part.

19 Early evidence indicates that harmful consequences of psychotherapists in California observing duties under the *Tarasoff* decision are imperceptible; see Wise (1978).

20 76 D.L.R. (3d) 688 (S.C.C.).

21 R.S.O. 1980, c. 262, s. 63. At the time, the provision was Section 59 of the Mental Health Act, R.S.O. 1970, c. 269.

22 See note 20, p. 692, per Laskin, C. J. C.

23 Compatibly with this principle, an Ontario county court declined to find that acupuncture constitutes ''the practice of medicine,'' because it was shown that physicians in the province are not trained in acupuncture and do not profess this to be one of their general skills; see *R. v. Gaulin* (1981), 34 O.R. (2d) 195 (Ont. Co. Ct.), in which a nonphysician performing acupuncture was held to commit no offense against the Health Disciplines Act by practicing medicine when medically unqualified. This decision followed *R. v. Wong* (1979), 50 C.C.C. (2d) 162 (Alta. Prov. Ct.).

24 See note 12.

25 See Linden (1973, p. 32, n. 13, and p. 33); see also the rejection of the professional standard of information disclosure as decisive to determine negligence in the informing process in *Hopp v. Lepp* (1980), 112 D.L.R. (3d) 67, per C. J. C. Laskin, p. 80.

26 (1974), 519 P.2d 981 (S.C. Wash.). The effect of this decision was subsequently reversed by legislation in the state of Washington.

27 Courts rarely need to be definitive, because the issue in litigation is commonly whether a given practice is to be considered professionally improper, rather than whether a proper practice is inadequate to fulfill legal expectations.

28 The Mental Hospitals Act, R.S.O. 1960, c. 236, s. 1(m).

29 The Mental Health Act, 1967, S.O. 1967, c. 185, s. 8(1)(a).

30 See the Mental Health Act, R.S.O. 1970, c. 269, as amended by S.O. 1978, c. 50.

31 See note 21.

32 Ibid., Section 12.

33 Ibid., Section 14(3), subject to the attending physician's admitting the person as an involuntary patient under a certificate of involuntary admission, when the person may be detained for longer periods; see Section 14(4).

34 Ibid., Section 14(1)(c).

35 See also Wexter's (1979) article, ''Patients, Therapists, and Third Parties: The Victimological Virtues of Tarasoff.''

36 Wexler (1979, p. 166) extensively reviews victimology literature, including studies showing how often in domestic violence, until the moment of one partner's striking out, the roles of victim and offender are interchangeable.

37 R.S.C. 1970, c. C-34. All references to Criminal Code sections will hereafter be by section number only. For a general review and critique of Part 21, see Webster and Dickens (1983).

38 Section 687.

39 Sentence for high treason, treason, and first- and second-degree murder are set in other provisions of the Criminal Code.

40 Section 688.

41 Ibid.
42 Section 689(1).
43 Section 689(2).
44 Section 690(1), emphasis added; use of the word "shall," as opposed to "may," shows a mandatory duty binding on the judge.
45 Section 690(2).
46 If the offender fails or refuses to nominate a psychiatrist, the court shall nominate one on the offender's behalf; see Section 690(3).
47 See the discussion in *Tarasoff*; note 3, p. 354.
48 *Murel v. Baltimore City Criminal Court* (1972), 92 S.Ct. 2091, cited in *Tarasoff*; note 3, p. 354. Ennis and Litwack (1974) found that professional social workers and correctional officials made more accurate predictions of dangerousness than psychotherapists; see p. 712.
49 For evidence that psychiatrists make assessments on the basis of personal values rather than by employing professional judgment, see Greenland (1977). For a comparable study elsewhere, see Pfafflin (1979).
50 The decision to apply for a finding of dangerous offender status is not uniformly reached among prosecutors, and a proposal to make an application may be bought off in a plea bargain. See generally Verdun-Jones and Cousineau (1979).
51 See note 48 and accompanying text.
52 See note 43.
53 See the section on "dangerousness" as a legal status under "Public Policy in the Face of Clinical Unpredictability of Dangerousness."
54 See note 3, p. 340. At the commencement of the circumstances of the case, the police were in fact notified, and they briefly detained the patient.
55 These circumstances are not the same, of course, in that a mental health professional's reluctance to notify, due to unreliability of prediction, cannot be so justified after a patient was apparently engaged in a dangerous act.
56 The *Tarasoff* court compatibly observed that "in this risk-infested society we can hardly tolerate the further exposure to danger that would result from a concealed knowledge of the therapist that his patient was lethal. . . . The containment of such risks lies in the public interest"; see note 3, pp. 347–8.
57 *Solicitor-General of Canada v. Royal Commission of Inquiry into Confidentiality of Health Records in Ontario* (1981), 128 D.L.R. (3d) 193 (S.C.C.), pp. 214– 15.
58 Formerly known as "Crown privilege."
59 See note 57, per Martland, J. p. 225.
60 A national voluntary quasi-public agency comparable to Canadian Children's Aid Societies.
61 *D. v. National Society for Prevention of Cruelty to Children,* [1978] A.C. 171, per Lord Simon of Glaisdale, p. 233.
62 See note 57, p. 226; ordinary legal defenses may protect disclosures to police, however, such as qualified privilege of nonmalicious communication made to an appropriately interested person.
63 (1980), 634 F.2d 650. This decision of the U. S. Court of Appeals for the First Circuit was remanded for retrial by the U. S. Supreme Court in its decision of June 18, 1982, under the name *Mills v. Rogers*, 102 S.Ct. 2442 (1982).
64 The constitutional provisions in question, notably the Fourteenth Amendment to the U.S. Constitution, have been introduced to Canada under the 1982 Canadian Charter of Rights and Freedoms, Section 7 of which governs "the right to life, liberty and security of the person and the right not to be deprived thereof except in accordance with the principles of fundamental justice."
65 A patient involuntarily detained on grounds of dangerousness is not necessarily incompetent to give or refuse consent to therapy; see *Rogers v. Okin,* note 63.
66 Treatment is therapeutically intended and is distinguishable from observation, examination, and restraint. Under Ontario's Mental Health Act (see note 21), "restrain" means "keep under con-

trol by the minimal use of such force, mechanical means or chemicals as is reasonable having regard to the physical and mental condition of the patient''; see section 1(t).

67 Notably *Addington v. Texas* (1979), 441 U.S. 418 (U.S.S.C.).

68 See note 63, p. 657.

69 See the section on involuntary civil committal under ''Public Reliance on Professional Prediction of Dangerousness.''

70 See note 63, p. 659.

71 The court observed (note 63, p. 661), ''Following a determination of incompetency, state actions based on *parens patriae* interests must be taken with the aim of making treatment decisions as the individual himself would were he competent to do so.''

72 See note 63, p. 656.

73 Ibid.

74 See *Cooper v. The Queen* (1980), 51 C.C.C. (2d) 129 (S.C.C.), especially the discussion of Dickson, J., p. 143.

75 (1979), 409 A.2d 1349, p. 1351.

76 Note the emphasis given to repetitive and patterned past behavior in Part 21 of the Criminal Code of Canada, concerning dangerous offenders; see text between notes 40 and 41.

77 See text and accompanying reference at note 9.

78 In *State v. Hudson* in New Hampshire, it was noted in the discussion of dangerousness as a legal condition that ''it has long been recognized in this State that even the condition of insanity may be proved by lay witnesses . . . and lay testimony has recently been held to satisfy Federal Constitutional standards''; see note 75, p. 1351.

79 See note 21.

80 See note 33.

81 By Section 10(4), the order directs and authorizes that the person be taken within 7 days to an appropriate place for assessment.

82 ''A review board shall be composed of three or five members, at least one and not more than two of whom are psychiatrists and at least one and not more than two of whom are barristers and solicitors and at least one of whom is not a psychiatrist or a barrister and solicitor''; see note 21, Section 30(2).

83 The 1978 amendments to the Mental Health Act (see note 30, Section 11) provided for appeals from review board decision to county or district courts; these provisions were proclaimed in force with effect from March 1, 1984.

84 This supposes that intervention with persons on an involuntary basis may itself be justifiable; for another view, see Morse (1982).

85 See generally Allen (1953, pp. 61–6) and Power (1981).

86 The statute of 34 Edw. III.

87 For its history and application, see Allen (1953) and Williams (1967, p. 87–113).

88 See note 37.

89 Section 745(2)–(4).

90 Section 746.

91 R.S.O. 1980, c. 66. Individual section references to provisions of the act will not be given later.

92 A family court may be appropriate, because of the issues and evidence that may be presented and because a court can be convened with great speed and in any suitable place.

93 Compare judicial powers under the Criminal Code, Section 465, 543 and, for instance, 738.

94 Force may be defensible in civil and criminal law under doctrines of necessity to save life. Criminal law may also accommodate a defense of mistake of fact, by which defendants must be judged as if what they (falsely) believed to be true was true. Civil proceedings for negligence might be resisted by evidence of observance of an appropriate standard of care, and necessity might resist claims for trespass to property and perhaps to the person. See Isenberg (1978).

95 On the definition of ''restraint,'' see note 66.

96 Compare the present law, which requires mental assessment within 120 hours; see text at note 33. The Mental Health Act intends assessment within 120 consecutive hours, rather than "five days," because a legal "day" is defined by reference to parts of days and when a "day" commences, and may exclude Sundays and certain public holidays.

97 Discussed in the section on involuntary civil committal under "Public Reliance on Professional Prediction of Dangerousness."

98 A person found incompetent to consent could be protected by an approved surrogate and by the court itself regarding risk-bearing treatments including drugs.

99 The question of standards of proof involved in commitment proceedings is discussed by Neff (1982).

100 See notes 57 and 61.

101 Section 178.23. By Section 178.23(2), disclosure provisions do not apply in the case of a warrant to intercept authorized under the Official Secrets Act.

102 There are distinctions, of course, regarding whether an individual must take an initiative to have a record disclosed or whether the record keeper has a duty of informing those recorded.

103 See note 91.

104 It has occasionally been argued that receipt of such notice can lead to improvement of child protection and of harmful adult behavior, so functioning as a contributory factor in therapy and prevention.

105 *Report of the Commission of Inquiry into the Confidentiality of Health Information* (Toronto: Government publisher, Ontario, 1980), recommendations 82–85, Chap. 23.

106 See note 21, Section 29(5).

107 Comparable protection against deprivation of liberty without due process now exists under the Canadian Charter of Rights and Freedoms; see note 64.

108 See note 63, p. 656.

109 Ibid., p. 657. The court had already urged the lower court to be creative in designing appropriate procedural mechanisms.

References

Allen, C. K. *The Queen's peace*. London: Stevens, 1953.

Ash, P. The reliability of psychiatric diagnosis. *Journal of Abnormal and Social Psychology*, 1949, *44*, 272–6.

Bergman, B. Z. Is the cloth unraveling? A first look at clergy malpractice. *San Fernando Valley Law Review*, 1981, *9*, 47–66.

Braley, N. B. Estelle v. Smith and psychiatric testimony: New limits on predicting future dangerousness. *Baylor Law Review*, 1981, *33*, 1015–34.

Curran, W. J., & Harding, T. W. *The law and mental health: Harmonizing objectives*. Geneva: World Health Organization, 1978.

Dershowitz, A. The psychiatrists' power in civil commitment: A knife that cuts both ways. *Psychology Today*, 1969, *2*, 42–7.

Diamond, B. L. The psychiatric prediction of dangerousness. *University of Pennsylvania Law Review*, 1974, *123*, 439–52.

Dickens, B. M. (1978). Legal protection of psychiatric confidentiality. *International Journal of Law and Psychiatry*, 1978, *1*, 255–81.

Dix, G. E. Participation by mental health professionals in capital murder sentencing. *International Journal of Law and Psychiatry*, 1978, *1*, 283–308.

Ennis, B. J., & Litwack, T. R. Psychiatry and the presumption of expertise: Flipping coins in the courtroom. *California Law Review*, 1974, *62*, 693–752.

Ericsson, S. E. Clergyman malpractice: Ramifications of a new theory. *Valparaiso University Law Review*, 1981, *16*, 163–84.

Fleming, J. G., & Maximov, B. The patient or his victim: The therapist's dilemma. *California Law Review*, 1974, *62*, 1025–68.

Glaser, D. The efficacy of alternative approaches to parole prediction. *American Sociological Review*, 1955, *20*, 283–7.

Greenland, C. Psychiatry and the dangerous sexual offender. *Canadian Psychiatric Association Journal*, 1977, *22*, 155–9.

Hunter, R., & Macalpine, I. *Three hundred years of psychiatry, 1535–1860*. London: Oxford University Press, 1963.

Isenberg, R. Medical necessity as a defense to criminal liability: *U.S.* v. *Randall*. *George Washington Law Review*, 1978, *46*, 273–98.

Kjervik, D. K. The psychiatric nurse's duty to warn potential victims of homicidal psychotherapy outpatients. *Law, Medicine and Health Care*, 1981, *9*(6), 11–16.

Klein, J. F. The dangerousness of dangerous offender legislation: Forensic folklore revisited. *Canadian Journal of Criminology and Corrections*, 1976, *18*, 109–22.

Kozol, H. L. Boucher, R. J., & Garofalo, R. F. The diagnosis and treatment of dangerousness. *Crime and Delinquency*, 1972, *18*,(4) 371–92.

Linden, A. M. The negligent doctor *Osgoode Hall Law Journal*, 1973, *11*, 31–9.

Morse, S. J. A preference for liberty: The case against involuntary commitment of the mentally disordered. *California Law Review*, 1982, *70*, 54–106.

Neff, Jr., R. C. Police power commitments: Towards a legal response to violence among the mentally ill. *University of Toledo Law Review*, 1982, *13*, 421–61.

Pfäfflin, F. The contempt of psychiatric experts for sexual convicts (Hamburg, Germany). *International Journal of Law and Psychiatry*, 1979, *2*, 485–97.

Picard, E. *Legal liability of doctors and hospitals in Canada*. Toronto: Carswell, 1978.

Power, P. ''An honour and a most singular one'': A review of the justices' preventive jurisdiction. *Monash University Law Review*, 1981, *8*, 69–133.

Price, R. R. ''Psychiatry, criminal-law reform and the 'mythophilic' impulse: On Canadian proposals for the control of the dangerous offender. *Ottawa Law Review*, 1970, *4*, 1–61.

Report of the Commission of Inquiry into the Confidentiality of Health Information. Toronto: Government Publisher, Ontario, 1980.

Schiffer, M. E. *Mental disorder and the criminal trial process*. Toronto: Butterworths, 1978.

Webster, C. D., & Dickens, B. M. *Deciding dangerousness: Policy alternatives for dangerous offenders*. Ottawa: (Federal) Ministry of Justice, 1983.

Weissbourd, R. Involuntary commitment: The move toward dangerousness. *John Marshall Law Review*, 1982, *15*, 83–113.

Wexler, D. B. Patients, therapists, and third parties: The victimological virtues of Tarasoff. *International Journal of Law and Psychiatry*, 1979, *2*, 1–28.

Wexler, D. B. *Mental health law and major issues*. New York: Plenum Books, 1981.

Williams, D. *Keeping the peace: The police and public order*. London: Hutchinson, 1967.

Wise, T. P. Where the public peril begins: A survey of psychotherapists to determine the effects of Tarasoff. *Stanford Law Review*, 1978, *31*, 165–90.

Verdun-Jones, S. N., & Cousineau, F. D. Cleaning the Augean Stables: A critical analysis of recent trends in the plea bargaining debate in Canada. *Osgoode Hall Law Journal*, 1979, *17*, 227–60.

12 Clinical predictors on trial: a case for their defense

Virginia J. McFarlane

The battle lines in the debate over the clinical prediction of dangerousness are drawn at the start of this volume. First, Professor Stone argues that, on the basis of present scientific knowledge, mental health professionals have no proper claim to expert status in this domain. Then, Professor Greenland, who admits the woeful lack of strong evidence to support the idea that clinicians can do the job expected of them by the courts, argues forcefully that psychiatrists and other mental health workers could, if they applied themselves to the task, demonstrate a capacity for accomplishing the predictive task in question. All the other contributors range between these two poles. Professor Dickens, although working from a broad legal perspective, finds himself more or less allied with Alan Stone and almost seems to take some pleasure in warning clinicians about the perils of making claims they cannot substantiate. Professor Dietz joins Cyril Greenland's camp in his quest for a way of limiting and defining the predictive question, possibly through the use of typologies. In the middle, several contributors deal with the dimensions of the scientific task and, in some cases, offer new data (Haynes, Martin, Dutton, Menzies, Webster, & Sepejak, and Steadman).

Although editors of a book of this kind might think that the reader has got to "come down" where he or she thinks best, there seems nonetheless to be some value in offering a conclusory comment. This chapter originated in a course on psychological aspects of criminal law, during which it was "suggested" to me by my professor, the senior editor of this volume, that I might read Monahan (1981), the draft manuscript of the present volume, and various other articles. I agreed to do this and, in addition, took on the experience of attending most of a hearing under Part 21 of the Criminal Code of Canada. This part deals with so-called dangerous offenders (see Webster & Dickens, 1983); it requires that at least one psychiatrist testify for the defense and one for the prosecution. A finding of dangerousness normally results in an indeterminant sentence. Sitting through this testimony made me realize that, given the present legal arrangements in Canada, which are not greatly different from those elsewhere (e.g., Sleffel, 1977), the clinician and indeed the social scientist, despite all of the uncertainties, must take a position on that continuum mentioned earlier. No matter how nice the legal analysis, no matter how penetrating and thorough the scientific thinking, in the end a decision has to be made with respect to that man or woman, that defendant, whose life hangs so precariously in the balance and who watches so anxiously as both sides do their utmost to convince the judge of one view or the other. Under the prevailing law, the issue has to be dealt with, and clinicians, whether they like it or not, currently must play some part in the deliberations in a wide range of jurisdictions. And just as the individual case has to be settled, no matter how uneasily or how unsatisfactorily, so too must the general issue of clinical predictive acumen be resolved, at least for a period. It was with these thoughts in mind that I wrote this summary chapter. The reader will see that the chapter attempts to capitalize on the courtroom drama. One side is pitted against the other to make the debate more interesting and to extend some of the issues outlined by other contributors in previous chapters. An additional reason for proceeding in this way is that it may tempt lawyers and mental health workers on either side of the issue in a particular case to make practical use of the scholarly material contained in this book. In a way, the chapter, with its frequent reference to foregoing contributions, serves as a kind of general index.

The case before the court

In this volume, Stone and Dickens forcefully remind the reader that mental health professionals'[1] predictions of dangerous behavior have been under attack for the past 20 years (see also Szasz, 1968). The first attack bombarded clinicians with "arguments" and "proofs" that they have no ability to assess and predict dangerousness. The second attack assailed them with "claims" and "evidence" that their expert testimony in court confuses the courts and obstructs the due process of law. Although the second attack was concerned mainly with pushing clinicians out of the courtroom, the first attack was an attempt to push them out of the prediction business altogether. So much criticism has been leveled at the predictive efforts of clinicians that it is time to hear what can be said in their favor. In this chapter, a case is presented for the defense of mental health professionals as predictors of dangerousness and as expert witnesses of the same. If at times the assertions and conclusions seem dogmatic, overly optimistic, and a trifle naive, it is only because I wish to stress the other side of this issue.

Court is in session

The defendants, mental health professionals, are charged with fraud and obstructing the due process of law. They are accused of rendering assessments and predictions of dangerousness, for which they have no expertise, and of offering such false assessments and predictions as expert testimony to courts of law. The defendants plead not guilty to both charges. We shall now hear from the prosecution with respect to the first charge.

Prosecution

In a haughty, self-assured tone of voice the prosecutor says: "Study after study in the past twenty years has demonstrated that mental health professionals are 'accurate in no more than one out of three predictions of violent behavior' " (Monahan, 1981, p. 77) "and that they overpredict dangerousness, yielding false positive rates of 60 percent and higher" (Cocozzo & Steadman, 1976; Kozol, Boucher, & Garofalo, 1972; State of Maryland, 1978; Thornberry & Jacoby, 1979). "These claims are not at all surprising," he continues, "when we consider the enormous and numerous difficulties inherent in the prediction of dangerousness and the ways in which clinicians go about the task." The prosecutor then plunges into his case, speaking at great length and bringing forth witnesses. I shall summarize his case, minus the rhetorical flourishes and innuendo.

Without the guidance of a standardized, systematic procedure that includes an operationalized definition of dangerousness and without clear and specific instructions as to what the court wants, clinicians must predict whether an individual will be dangerous over the next several years. Long-term predictions are especially difficult to make because the future living conditions (e.g., prison, hospital, or community) are unknown and will be determined in part by the very clinical prediction itself. Even in the absence of these inherent complications, predicting dangerous behavior would be difficult because dangerous behavior has such a low base rate of occurrence.

Furthermore, clinicians hinder prediction accuracy. Typically, they use only a few sources of information, placing too much emphasis on police reports, diagnoses, and intuition and not enough on situational factors and base-rate information when it is available. Several idiosyncratic factors (e.g., disciplinary orientation) and social interactional factors (e.g., wanting to appear "expertly sensible") also affect the reliability and validity of predictions (Pfohl, 1978). As well, there is no mechanism whereby the courts can inform clinicians of their "hits" and "misses" (Webster & Dickens, 1983). Without this kind of information, it would be essentially impossible for a clinician to evaluate and improve his or her prediction accuracy (Webster, 1984).

The research claims that clinicians are poor predictors of dangerousness has led many critics to question whether they should be the ones to do the job (e.g., Dietz in chapter 6). In an American case in 1975, the judge said:

It may legitimately be inquired whether there is anything in the education, training, or experience of psychiatrists which renders them particularly adept at predicting dangerous behavior. . . . there is a growing consensus that psychiatrists are not uniquely qualified to predict dangerous behavior and are in fact less accurate in their predictions than other professionals (*People v. Burnick,* 1975, cited in Schiffer, 1982, p. 276).

Martin in chapter 5 notes that "psychiatrists are trained to diagnose and treat treatable mental disorder, which most often is not associated with physically dangerous behavior." Dix (1980) has argued that their "skills in identifying, prognosticating, and treating serious mental illness" do not necessarily indicate an ability to predict the dangerous behavior of those not "exhibiting symptoms of such illness" (p. 528). Dix (1980) has also argued that the professional orientation of clinicians predisposes them to overpredict. In their diagnostic practice, pathological findings can lead to unnecessary treatment, which to them is preferable to not detecting a pathological condition and failing to provide needed treatment. Dix claims that this attitude may carry over to situations in which they are called on to predict dangerousness.

Mental health professionals themselves also seem to be questioning whether they should continue to proffer predictions. (The prosecution is trying to show here that the guilty consciences of mental health professionals are further evidence of their complicity.) In an American study, several hundred practicing psychiatrists, clinical psychologists, and mental health lawyers estimated predictive accuracy to be between 40 and 46% (Kahle & Sales, 1980). P. Hillen and C. D. Webster (in Webster & Dickens, 1983) similarly found that the majority of Canadian psychiatrists, lawyers, and research- or treatment-oriented professionals whom they questioned estimated predictions to be at chance, or a little better than chance, levels. Hillen and Webster were "struck by the fact that Canadian psychiatrists appear to think that they are being forced by law into offering opinions of dubious quality" (in Webster & Dickens, 1983, p. 46).

The prosecutor concludes his case by quoting Alan Stone (chapter 1):

Psychiatrists and others who appear in court to offer predictions of violence allow the courts to continue to deny that they have one foot in quicksand. This in the long run is a disservice to the law and to the attempts to establish psychiatry and psychology as scientific disciplines.

Defense

The defense counsel rises and, in an equally haughty and self-assured tone, says: "The attacks on the accuracy of predictions of violence have indeed been fierce. Clinicians have been bombarded with "proofs" of their inability to predict. It is hardly surprising that they *appear* to be disclaiming any predictive expertise; they have their backs to the wall. They would *appear* to be fools if they did not occasionally concede and surrender. They would not, however, *be* fools. And they would only *appear* to be fools to those who overlook, or simply cannot see, the serious conceptual and methodological flaws of the prediction research.'' At this point, the defense counsel plunges into a lengthy discourse and presentation of witnesses. I shall summarize his comments and those of his witnesses as I did for the prosecution.

Stone (chapter 1) ''found the published studies of prediction woefully inadequate, poorly conceived, wrongly interpreted, and well below any acceptable standard of scientific research or even solid clinical experience.'' Examples of the flaws of the prediction research indicate that the conclusion that clinicians have no capacity to predict dangerousness may be unwarranted. The follow-up intervals have been too short to test predictive accuracy fully. That is, if the intervals had been longer, more individuals may have been found to be violent (Menzies et al., chapter 8). The number of individuals found to be violent may have also been underestimated because of a failure to ''triangulate follow-up assaultiveness, by concatenating official data, self-reports, and victimization analysis,'' and by a failure to include reports of violence in mental health institutions (Menzies et al., chapter 8). Most of the studies lack external validity because they deal with selective subject populations (Menzies et al., chapter 8). For example, failure to predict the violent behavior of mentally ill subjects (e.g., Quinsey, Pruesse, & Fernley 1975; Steadman & Cocozza, 1974; Thornberry & Jacoby, 1979) does not tell us about clinicians' abilities to predict the behavior of non-mentally ill subjects (Dix, 1980, p. 532). Furthermore, because comprehensive assessments were rarely done (Dietz, chapter 6), the studies are unable to ''provide reliable evidence bearing upon the predictive value of careful assessments by a skilled clinician'' (Dix, 1980, p. 533). The English Floud committee (1981) stated that these studies ''provide better evidence of bad practice than of the state of the art of assessing dangerousness'' (Greenland, chapter 2). In other words, a critical examination of the prediction outcome research reveals that the capacity of mental health professionals to predict dangerousness has not yet been determined!

The recent and carefully executed research of Menzies et al. (chapter 8) suggests that mental health professionals may have some predictive capacity (see also Sepejak et al., 1983). These researchers obtained significantly positive correlations between predictions and outcome measures of violence. However, these correlations are very low; they

are severely limited by the context of the evaluation, the cross-sectional nature of the pretrial remand, the absence of criteria for operationalizing dangerousness, the failure of courts to provide feedback to the clinic, and the inattention to contextual or situational determinants of dangerous behavior.

Considering these difficulties, as well as others, it is actually surprising that their correlation coefficients are as high as they are and that they are significant. It may be that these methodological difficulties, which will probably hold for any research endeavors in the near future, result in an underestimation of clinicians' capacity to predict dangerous behavior. In other words, their capacity to predict may be better than research efforts can detect. This possibility should give pause to those who would abandon the use of clinical predictions of dangerous behavior. Reconsideration is further warranted by the finding of Menzies et al. that there are large individual differences in prediction accuracy, which may indicate that there are individuals who are relatively "good" at predicting dangerous behavior, especially when they are confronted with certain types of patients. If these individuals could be identified and the types of patients that they work best with specified, then perhaps future predictions of dangerousness could be limited to those with the greatest degree of expertise.

Abandonment of the use of clinical predictions of dangerousness has been argued, as noted earlier, on the grounds that there is nothing about clinicians' training and skills that would render them adept at such predictions and that may, on the contrary, actually cause them to overpredict dangerous behavior. Regarding the first argument, it is important to realize that it can also be said that

mental health professionals, by virtue of their skills in diagnosing and predicting the afflictions of abnormal people, have or develop similar skills regarding normal people. Further, it can be asserted that people who engage in antisocial behaviour are sufficiently 'abnormal' to come within mental health professionals' area of expertise, even if such individuals do not exhibit symptoms of traditional mental illness (Dix, 1980, p. 528).

John Monahan, in the past one of the most outspoken critics of clinical predictions, has suggested that clinical predictions may be particularly appropriate and valuable if used with caution, when rare events have to be taken into account and when short-term emergency predictions are required (Monahan, 1981).

Regarding the second argument, it is important to realize that there are profound social and political constraints that would account for overprediction, regardless of the predictor's training. These constraints place the predictor in a dilemma:

If he releases a rehabilitated man who shortly resumes his old pattern of crime, it reflects poorly on the entire profession and arouses public skepticism and indignation, especially since such cases are apt to be widely publicized and sensationalized. If he detains a man excessively long, he may have to deal with his own conscience, or he may undo his own rehabilitative efforts by encouraging feelings of hopelessness and betrayal in the inmate (Schiffer, 1982, p. 282).

Given the public outcry whenever released offenders have committed violent offenses, it would not be surprising if clinicians overpredicted, opting for public safety over the freedom of the individual offender.

Court in recess

During the first session of the trial, I outlined the case for the prosecution and for the defense with respect to the accusation that mental health professionals are poor predictors of dangerousness and that they should therefore cease to make such predictions. The prosecution's case rested on the grounds that empirical research indicates the validity of the accusation given the difficulty of the task, as well as clinicians' methods and lack of training for making such predictions. The defense's case rested on the grounds that the empirical research referred to by the prosecution is flawed and cannot determine clinicians' capacities to predict dangerousness; more recent research suggests that some individual clinicians may be relatively good at such predictions; most current research efforts are likely to underestimate capacities to predict; and clinicians' training may enhance their ability to predict dangerousness. The case for the defense, however, is not complete. If mental health professionals are going to continue to make predictions of dangerousness, they must show that the difficulties inherent in the task can be overcome and that their methods can be placed beyond reproach. This is what the defense attempts to accomplish in the next session of the trial. I have summarized some of the proposals that the defense counsel puts forth.

Defense case resumed

The criticism that mental health professionals use only a few sources of information can be easily redressed. Dietz (chapter 6) recommends more extensive interviews and investigations of the subject's criminal history. The defense argues that, despite the cost in time, effort, and dollars, a more thorough investigation is definitely worth the trouble because the stakes – an individual's freedom and the protection of society – are so high. The only problem that the defense sees is that an assessor would collect too much information and be unable to distinguish relevant from irrelevant data. As Haynes (chapter 4) notes, it is important to "distinguish between what is important to measure and what one can measure well." The defense suggests legislation that specifies exactly what sources of information the predicting clinician *must* use.

The defense also suggests legislation that specifies a standard procedure for assessing dangerousness. Martin's suggestions in chapter 5 for standardizing the diagnosis of psychiatric disorders could be applied to standardizing predictions of dangerousness. If certain behaviors and offenses were determined a priori to be more or less associated with future violence, then a prediction of the probability of future violence could be made and supported by examples of the individual's behavior and offenses. This requires that research be done to determine which behaviors and offenses are associated, and to what extent, with future violence. In other words, we need to determine the predictor variables of future violence. Dietz (chapter 6) has taken the first step in research of this type by listing several characteristics, behaviors, and offenses as possible predictor variables. Unfortunately, identifying predictor variables and calculating their probabilities would leave many problems unresolved. For example, how should probabilities be combined with one another, and how should they be viewed in light of findings from other sources, such as psychological tests? Nevertheless, because predictor variables are more or less factual; they would, it is to be hoped, lead to predictions that are more objective than current predictions. They would also lead to predictions made in probabilistic terms. At present, predictions are made in terms of personality traits. That is, the clinician will state that the offender is or is not a dangerous person. But dangerousness is not necessarily an enduring quality. Whether or not an individual will be dangerous changes from time to time and place to place. Hence, predictions can only, and should only, be made in probabilistic terms. This point has been made by several researchers (e.g., Monahan, 1981; Webster & Dickens, 1983; Haynes, chapter 4; Martin, chapter 5).

Several researchers have also made the point that prediction would be greatly enhanced if clinicians critically appraised themselves and their predictive decision making. With respect to self-appraisal, Dietz (chapter 6) recommends that predicting clinicians "articulate their assumptions and underlying beliefs" so as to avoid making "illusory correlations" (Monahan, 1981, p. 62). Clinicians becoming aware of their subjectivity would certainly be taking the first step toward objectivity. They would also be taking the first step toward putting themselves in "another person's shoes." Webster and Ben-Aron (chapter 3) suggest that "clinicians must surely use themselves as the microscope." Only if they know their own frailties and shortcomings can they understand and come to terms with others. Although appraising their predictive decision making would be facilitated by reports from the courts regarding "hits" and "misses," the present absence of such reports is no excuse for failing to undertake such measurement ventures in the future. Clinicians must simply track down this information – violent behavior – from the courts, correctional institutions, and hospitals. Without this return of information, predictive decision making cannot improve and will continue to "hide behind a screen of 'professional judgment' " (Monahan, 1981, p. 40).

Prosecution interjection

After listening patiently to the defense's rather lengthy discourse, the prosecutor objects, saying: "The defense's suggestions for improving clinical predictions of dangerousness are all very well, but they are rather scattered and unintegrated. If mental health professionals are going to continue predicting dangerousness, then I suggest they must demonstrate that they have some kind of comprehensive method for doing so – a model, if you please. The defense's ramblings indicate that they are far from achieving this."

Defense reply

"On the contrary!" the defense counsel retorts. "I was just about to lay down my trump card." The defense then proceeds to describe John Monahan's model for predicting dangerousness, pointing out how it holds the possibility of overcoming many of the difficulties inherent in the task and placing the methods of mental health professionals beyond reproach. He explains that Monahan's model for predicting violent behavior consists of 12 questions that address such issues as personal competence, ethical concerns, kinds of information to be gathered, methods for gathering the information, and the reliability and validity of the information. Instead of summarizing the defense counsel's rather detailed description of Monahan's model, I refer you to Mr. Monahan himself (Monahan, 1981, chapter 6).

Prosecution reply

The prosecutor has heard enough about Monahan's questions. "This model by Mr. Monahan is not going to resolve *all* of the problems of predicting dangerousness! Nor is it going to place the methods of clinicians beyond reproach! The necessary information is not always available, as the defense has conceded. And even if it were, the clinician still has a tremendous amount of interpretive discretion at his or her disposal. What if the clinician were afraid of the offender during the course of the assessment? And what if the clinician were really more concerned with being deemed an 'expert' than in being expert about his or her job?"

Defense reply

"Of course, there are sources of error that are difficult, if not impossible to eliminate," replies the defense counsel. "Videotaping the assessment interview, however, would help to control some of the problems the prosecutor has so astutely pointed out. It would also serve as a check that the standard procedure had been followed. If bias were detected, the court could rule the evidence inadmissible or weigh it less heavily. Certainly, the plan is not perfect. It has to be implemented, tested, and revised accordingly. A tremendous amount of research must be done if we are to minimize prediction errors. And this is the point: All that we can ever hope to do is minimize errors! We will never eliminate them. If we demand that predictions meet stringent requirements, then we will have fewer false positives, but only at the price of more false negatives. Conversely, if we broaden the requirements for positive predictions, then we will have fewer false negatives and more false positives. The requirements should be decided by the courts and legislature – clinicians don't dispute this. But you will always have error, regardless of who does the predicting'' (Webster & Dickens, 1983).

Prosecution interjection

"Regardless of who does the predicting?" the prosecutor jeers. "You have just undermined your own argument. If there are always going to be mistakes, then let's have legal people making them. There's no need for confusing the issue further by bringing in mental health people."

Defense statement

"That's where *you* are wrong," the defense counsel snaps back. "It is mental health people who are, and have long been, entrusted by the law with this task. The law is very slow to change. And why should it change? What are the alternatives? There is no empirical 'proof' that any other group, professional or otherwise, has more skill than mental health professionals at predicting dangerousness. And even if there were 'proof,' I submit that the law would be well advised to be wary of it and continue to walk 'a respectful distance behind science' " (Haward, 1976, p. 313).

Court adjourns

The court has finished dealing with the first charge and will defer judgment until it has dealt with the second charge. The third session of the trial opens with the judge reminding the court that it is here to determine whether mental health professionals are guilty of obstructing the due process of law.

Prosecution

The prosecutor rises, adjusts his robes, clears his throat, and in a very somber tone begins: "The court is here today to deal with a very grave concern to us all. The courts have been thrown into chaos, the adversary system has been usurped, and the rule of law and trier of fact have been overrun by clinicians presenting their 'expert' testimony of predictions of dangerousness."

"The difficulties in evaluating this 'expert' testimony are manifold," he continues. "The abstruse nature of psychiatry and the compiling of data by subjective methods that are not easily explained to others and are not open to cross-examination because the courts receive only the results without any reference to the methods by which they were obtained – these are obstacles that the court must overcome if it is to evaluate, cross-examine, predictions of dangerousness.

Cross-examination is limited by the code of confidentiality that exists between the clinician and the patient. And it is next to impossible to evaluate this testimony when there is no standard procedure for giving it. The court cannot even determine if the clinicians' definition of dangerous behavior is even remotely similar to that of the court'' (Needell, 1980). ''Parenthetically, I wonder if the adversary system is at all suited to the dispassionate presentation of data in the hope of arriving at 'psychiatric truth' '' (Needell, 1980).

''This brings me to my next point: The rendering of 'expert' predictions of dangerous behavior by clinicians opens the door to corruption of the court. Besides the more obvious corruptions of each counsel bringing in the 'best witness' for his or her case'' (Needell, 1980) ''and the rather lucrative rewards for clinicians doing as they are bid, there are other, more subtle corruptions. Offering predictions of dangerousness to the courts provides clinicians with the opportunities of enhancing their self-image as an expert and of publically expounding and propagandizing their latest pet theories'' (Yarmey, 1979). ''Furthermore, clinicians don't make professional or scientific statements concerning an individual's behavior. They say 'Mr. X is too dangerous to be released.' This is a legal, moral, or social value judgment. The courts are being controlled by the personal values of mental health professionals!'' (Fersch, 1980). ''Indeed, there is empirical support for this notion.'' The prosecutor then brings forth witnesses who testify that their research indicates that judges and juries rely heavily on clinicians' predictions of dangerousness, giving them far more weight than is warranted. I shall summarize their findings and interpretations.

Evidence of courts being highly influenced by clinicians' recommendations was found in British, American, and Canadian studies. In two British studies, the courts followed clinicians' recommendations for psychiatric treatment of the accused in 90% (Sparks, 1966) and 92% (De Berken, 1960) of the cases reviewed. Dershowitz (1978) found that in two of the three American studies that he examined, the judges relied heavily on clinicians' reports (cited in Dix, 1980, p. 578, n. 174). And more recently, Webster, Menzies, and Jackson (1982, appendix E) found that Canadian judges' dispositions were generally in accord with psychiatric recommendations, especially when custodial recommendations were made (agreement between recommendation and disposition was 73% in these cases).

Three reasons for this overreliance were put forth. One is that the scientific jargon (Webster & Dickens, 1983, p. 71) and the attractive manner in which clinicians present their evidence (Dix, 1980) impresses both judges and jurors. Another reason is that judges and jurors are influenced, and perhaps intimidated, by the scientific qualifications of the witness (Webster & Dickens, 1983). The third and most disturbing reason is that clinicians' testimony makes difficult decisions easier to make.

A jury often wants – indeed needs – to believe that the expert's opinion stems from his or her special abilities as a professional. . . . they want to believe that an individual who would do these horrible things is a different species from them. [The psychiatrist] tells them this person doesn't deserve to [be free.]² He makes a decision easier (Ewing, 1982, pp. 412–13).

Prins (1980) also found evidence suggesting that magistrates, as well as jurors, desire help with their decision making.

The upshot of all this is that mental health professionals are actually making decisions for the courts. This is not at all surprising. Clinicians do not understand the adversary system; they present conclusory testimony as if it were up to them to decide on the verdict (Parker, 1980). Indeed, Pfohl (1978) found that clinicians would write their reports to the court so as to try to control the outcome. For example, their diagnoses and predictions were occasionally based, not on what they believed they had found and believed to be true, but on what they thought would lead to the most appropriate disposition for the individual. The prosecutor asserts that this is clearly a usurpation of the adversary system, the rule of law, and the trier of fact. He protests that deciding that an individual is dangerous should be seen to be what it is, namely, "a sociopolitical judgment rather than a psychiatric diagnosis" (Greenland, chapter 2).

Prosecution's final argument

At this point the prosecutor smugly declares: "The courts do not need clinicians' predictions of dangerousness. There is evidence indicating that they base their predictions predominantly on police reports and intuition. Testimony based on these sources is not outside the experience and knowledge of judges and jurors, as it should be to qualify as expert testimony. I submit that the courts should abolish 'expert' predictions of dangerousness and get back to doing thorough criminal investigations and to making these difficult moral and social decisions. The courts should not stoop to having mental health professionals 'launder' their decisions for them (Monahan, 1981). We in the courts must stop 'using' mental health professionals to suit our own doubtful ends" (Appelbaum, 1984).

Defense

The defense counsel rises, shuffles his papers, looks up at the ceiling, and, speaking in an almost quiet voice, with just the appropriate hint of emotion which suggests that he is the last defender of a noble cause, says: "To abolish expert predictions of dangerousness would be to deny the courts one of their most valuable sources of evidence. This will be especially clear when I have shown how this testimony can be improved. If mental health professionals have failed to demonstrate an appreciation for the adversary system, it is because of the role that the courts have forced them into. The courts have erroneously and implicitly demanded that clinicians decide whether an individual is dangerous. Is it any wonder that they have done so? The criticisms made by the prosecution clearly call for standardization, regulation, and quality control of psychiatric testimony so that it is given its proper weighting and so that decision making is returned to the courts.'' The defense then proceeds to demonstrate how these goals could be achieved. The following is my summary of these proceedings.

The first step toward improving courtroom testimony would be to increase the level of communication between the law and psychiatry. The defense counsel cites H. R. Rollin as quoted by Menzies et al. in chapter 8:

> There must be far more communication between jurists and psychiatrists so that the strong arm of the law knows what the weak hand of psychiatry is doing, and even more important, perhaps, capable of doing. . . . Unless and until something of this sort is brought about, the Gilbertian situation which now obtains will continue, and psychiatrists and jurists, instead of being . . . brothers-in-law will become increasingly partners-in-crime.

Clinicians' ability to do the court's bidding would be enhanced if the courts stipulated guidelines for their reports, defined the legal status of their reports, dictated a policy to be followed concerning the disclosure of their findings to defense and Crown, and reported the judicial results of their efforts (Webster et al., 1982).

Several witnesses were called by the defense to suggest means of standardizing and regulating courtroom testimony. Their main points are summarized in what follows. First, clinicians would have to meet stringent criteria to qualify as experts. They would have to demonstrate, for example, that they had spent a given number of years working as mental health professionals and a certain number of years working in forensic settings. As well, and this is most important, would-be experts would have to demonstrate knowledge of probability theory and basic statistical concepts (see Dix, 1980).

Second, they would be permitted to present evidence only of a given, controlled quality. For example, predictions could be made only in probabilistic and not conclusory terms (Monahan, 1981) and only if they were substantiated by a thorough and objective assessment that would have to be fully described (or even demonstrated by videotape). Clinicians would also have to state their personal value assumptions (Fersch, 1980) by answering a series of standard questions that would have been found empirically to tap such basic beliefs. This precaution would, it is hoped, prevent clinicians from imposing their values on the court. Another precaution would be not to allow a clinician to make a prediction without the court also hearing from another clinician, a criminologist perhaps, about the problems inherent in the task of predicting dangerousness (Webster & Dickens, 1983). At present, courts occasionally request this type of testimony for dangerous offender hearings.

Third, a clearly prescribed procedure for the presentation of expert predictions would have to be enforced. This procedure could easily be based on Monahan's (1981) model for assessing dangerousness, with a few revisions to adapt it to the courtroom. Psychiatric evidence would have to cover specific questions that would have been decided upon a priori. Most important, whatever procedure were decided upon, the concept of dangerousness would have to be explicitly defined, operationalized, and made known to clinicians and the courts. Positive predictions would then depend on whether or not an individual met the criteria for dangerousness that had been decided upon a priori. Having a clearly prescribed procedure would provide for cross-examining and weighing the evidence. Having to follow a procedure would, it is hoped, reduce the opportunity for clinicians to capitalize on the hearing or trial to enhance their reputations or to promote their latest theories. Furthermore, this procedure could be part of a larger procedure, which would include tapping several sources of information to determine dangerousness. For example, correctional officers, hospital staff, and various other character witnesses could be called on to assist the courts in making these arduous decisions (Dix, 1980; Pfohl, 1978).

Needell (1980) has recommended two schemes, either of which would satisfy the need for quality control of expert testimony in the courtroom. His first scheme consists of substituting a panel composed of a judge, lawyer, and psychiatrist for the jury (or for a single judge, as the case may be). Each member of the panel would be allowed to question the expert witness directly. "Because a psychiatrist presumably is better able to understand the subtleties and ramifications of psychiatric testimony than is a judge, this plan would considerably strengthen the court's ability to identify bias and inaccuracy" (Needell, 1980, p. 440). In addition, it would not be too costly, nor would it be difficult to implement and administer because its format is already known to legal and medical people for screening malpractice and personal injury cases.

According to Needell's second scheme, the court would appoint an independent expert (psychiatrist or psychologist) in addition to those provided by the defense and prosecution. This expert would testify as any other, rendering substantiated predictions of dangerousness and being subject to examination and cross-examination by both parties. The court-appointed expert would not be allied to either party and therefore would feel free to maintain an independent view. "Hence, he or she [would] be able to discuss dispassionately the possible theories that could explain the behavior at issue, even while advocating the theory he or she prefers" (Needell, 1980, p. 443). It is doubtful that juries would assume that the independent expert's testimony was infallable, thereby being unduly influenced by it. In cases in which court-appointed experts have been used, this has not happened (see Needell, 1980, 93, 94). Needell lists three factors that would mitigate concern about the influence of a court-appointed expert: (a) Both parties would be able to cross-examine the witness on the merits of his or her testimony; (b) both parties would be able to challenge his or her competency; and (c) it would not be totally undesirable if jurors lent a court-appointed expert extra credence, because he or she would be impartial and likely to provide the most accurate and bias-free testimony. This scheme would guarantee against bias through the "impartial character of the court-appointed expert" (Needell, 1980, p. 444), and it would guarantee against inaccuracy through the stringent criteria for qualifying as a court-appointed expert. In addition, an impartial expert would expose the experts for the defense and Crown to criticism, which "would strongly encourage them to take greater care in proffering testimony" (Needell, 1980, p. 445).

By the standardization and quality control of expert testimony, it is likely that decision making will naturally return to the courts. Be that as it may, Dickens (chapter 11) proposes "(a) that 'dangerousness' be recognized as a legal status as opposed to a psychiatric condition and (b) that dangerousness be determined by due process of law in an adequately conducted hearing." By recognizing dangerousness as a legal status in the same way that "insanity" and "disease of the mind" are recognized, it would, according to Dickens, have a substantial medical component, requiring expert medical witnesses, but its "nature and basis" would be determined by a judge or jury. And this, Dickens says, is as it should be because "any interference with the freedom of individuals and with their legal rights to autonomy and personal integrity can be justified only as an outcome of determinations made in accordance with due process of law."

The third session of the trial ends with the court having heard from both the prosecution and the defense with respect to the second charge, the obstruction of the due process of law. The trial resumes for the fourth and final session to hear the judge's verdict.

The verdict

The judge solemnly enters the court, settles himself comfortably in his chair, examines a document passed to him by the clerk, and then stares vacantly into space as the clerk of the court fills his water glass. He then rummages about among his papers and the large volumes that surround and shield him from the view of all but those who are sitting in the center of the court. Raising his eyes over the rims of his half-glasses, he peers out at the court and begins: "There is no doubt that, regardless of what is decided here today, 'dangerousness' [will] remain a 'dangerous concept' " (Scott, 1977). "Balancing individual freedom and the protection of society will still be extremely difficult and at times will be unfair to one or the other. Many other moral concerns will constantly demand attention. Some of these – whether or not predicting dangerousness is consistent with the clinicians' scientific and healing roles, for example – will best be dealt with by mental health professionals themselves (Ewing, 1982).

"Nevertheless, decisions as to whether certain individuals are dangerous must still be made. Society is adamant about this. In the past, courts have found it prudent to ask mental health professionals to *assist* them in this arduous task. The prosecution has informed us that their assistance hasn't always taken the form that it should have. Some of the prosecution's criticisms were shown to be without substance, whereas others were shown to be well founded. For example, we saw that the empirical research does not necessarily indicate that clinicians have no capacity for predicting dangerousness, and we also saw that judges and juries do rely too heavily on clinicians' predictions. However, there is hope that predicting dangerousness and rendering courtroom testimony of the same can be improved by implementing some of the proposals that the defense has so painstakingly described. (Of course, the ideal would be to prevent dangerous behavior altogether. And I must add that the defense has informed me that there are proposals addressing this issue [Dickens, chapter 11; Greenland, chapter 2].)

"It is my conviction that despite the criticisms, and in light of these promising proposals, mental health professionals are, and will be, the best individuals for the jobs of predicting dangerousness and rendering such predictions as expert testimony in court. I therefore find the defendants, mental health professionals, not guilty of either charge."

The case is closed.

Notes

1 The terms "mental health professional" and "clinician" refer here to psychiatrists and clinical psychologists, although occasionally they refer to social workers and nurses who work in forensic settings.
2 In the original this sentence read, "[The psychiatrist] tells them this person doesn't deserve to live." Because we do not have capital punishment in Canada, I changed the sentence for continuity purposes.

References

Appelbaum, P. S. The Supreme Court looks at psychiatry. *American Journal of Psychiatry,* 1984, *141,* 827–35.
Cocozza, J. J., & Steadman, H. J. The failure of psychiatric predictions of dangerousness: Clear and convincing evidence. *Rutgers Law Review,* 1976, *29,* 1084–1101.
De Berken, P. State of mind reports: The inadequate personality. *British Journal of Criminology,* 1960, *1,* 6–20.
Dix, G. E. Clinical evaluation of the "dangerousness" of "normal" criminal defendants. *Virginia Law Review,* 1980, *66,* 523–81.
Ewing, C. P. "Dr. Death" and the case for an ethical ban on psychiatric and psychological predictions of dangerousness in capital sentencing proceedings. *American Journal of Law and Medicine,* 1982, *8,* 407–28.

Fersch, E. A. *Psychology and psychiatry in courts and corrections: Controversy and change.* New York: Wiley, 1980.

Haward, L. R. C. Experimentation in forensic psychiatry. *Criminal Justice and Behavior,* 1976, *3,* 301–14.

Kahle, L., & Sales, B. Due process of law and the attitudes of professionals toward involuntary civil commitment. In P. Lipsitt & B. Sales (Eds.), *New directions in psychological research.* New York: Van Nostrand Reinhold, 1980.

Kozol, H., Boucher, R., & Garofalo, R. The diagnosis and treatment of dangerousness. *Crime and Delinquency,* 1972, *18,* 371–92.

Monahan, J. *Predicting violent behavior: An assessment of clinical techniques.* Beverly Hills: Sage, 1981.

Monahan, J. Clinical prediction of violent behavior. *Psychiatric Annals,* 1982, *12,* 509–13.

Needell, J. E. Psychiatric expert witnesses: Proposals for change. *American Journal of Law and Medicine,* 1980, *6,* 425–47.

Parker, L. C. Jr. *Legal psychology: eyewitness testimony: Jury behavior.* Springfield, Ill.: Thomas, 1980.

Pfohl, S. J. *Predicting dangerousness: The social construction of psychiatric reality.* Lexington, Mass.: Heath, 1978.

Prins, H. *Offenders, deviants or patients? An introduction to the study of socio-forensic problems.* London: Tavistock, 1980.

Quinsey, V. L., Pruesse, M., & Fernley, R. Oak Ridge patients: Prerelease characteristics and postrelease adjustment. *Journal of Psychiatry and Law,* Spring 1975, pp. 63–77.

Schiffer, M. E. *Psychiatry behind bars: A legal perspective.* Toronto: Butterworths, 1982.

Scott, P. D Assessing dangerousness in criminals. *British Journal of Psychiatry,* 1977, *131,* 127–42.

Sepejak, D. S., Menzies, R. J., Webster, C. D., & Jensen, F. A. S. Clinical predictions of dangerousness: Two-year follow-up of 408 pre-trial forensic cases. *American Academy of Psychiatry and the Law,* 1983, *11,* 171–81.

Sleffel, L. *The law and the dangerous criminal: Statutory attempts at definition and control.* Lexington, Mass.: Heath, 1977.

Sparks, R. F. The decision to remand for mental examination. *British Journal of Criminology,* 1966, *6,* 6–26.

State of Maryland. *Maryland's defective delinquency statute: A progress report.* Unpublished manuscript, Department of Public Safety and Correctional Services, 1978.

Steadman, H. J., & Cocozza, J. J. *Careers of the criminally insane: Excessive social control of deviance.* Lexington, Mass.: Heath, 1974.

Szasz, T. S. *Law, liberty, and psychiatry.* New York: MacMillan, 1968.

Thornberry, T. P. & Jacoby, J. *The criminally insane: A community follow-up of mentally ill offenders.* Chicago: University of Chicago Press, 1979.

Webster, C. D. How much of the clinical predictability of dangerousness issue is due to language and communication difficulties?: Some sample courtroom questions and some inspired but heady answers. *International Journal of Offender Therapy and Comparative Criminology,* 1984, *28,* 159–67.

Webster, C. D., & Dickens, B. *Deciding dangerousness: Policy alternatives for dangerous offenders.* Ottawa: Department of justice, 1983.

Webster, C. D., Menzies, R. J., Butler, B. T., & Turner, R. E. Forensic psychiatric assessment in selected Canadian cities. *Canadian Journal of Psychiatry,* 1982, *27,* 455–62.

Webster, C. D., Menzies, R. J., & Jackson, M. A. *Clinical assessment before trial: Legal issues and mental disorder.* Toronto: Butterworths, 1982.

Yarmey, A. D. *The psychology of eyewitness testimony.* New York: Free Press, 1979.

Author index

227

Subject index